Diet Secrets Every Person Must Know

by

Robert K. Christiansen

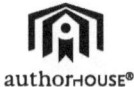

authorHOUSE®

AuthorHouse™
1663 Liberty Drive, Suite 200
Bloomington, IN 47403
www.authorhouse.com
Phone: 1-800-839-8640

First published by AuthorHouse 6/28/2007

ISBN: 978-1-4259-8690-2 (sc)

Library of Congress Control Number: 2006911041

Printed in the United States of America
Bloomington, Indiana

This book is printed on acid-free paper.

DIET SECRETS EVERY PERSON MUST KNOW

In opening, I must tell you, I am not a doctor, I am not an expert in nutrition, and I am certainly not your mother. I am an ordinary person just like you. The information you are about to read is purely my opinion.

When I was young I wanted to be president of the United States so I could make positive changes in people's lives. But I didn't come from a political family and realized that dream may be a stretch, so I decided to try to help the people in other ways. I was compelled to write this course on diet secrets after seeing so many people struggling with their weight (and I did, too, in my early years). I observed people close to me on diets for 20 years losing the same 5 pounds over and over and over but never reaching their goal to be slim and trim, trying one diet after another with little or no result. Trying the diet pills that would make you lose 10 pounds in the first week or the magic drink that would melt the pounds away or the exercise equipment that was a sure thing. Bottom line, if all of the products on the market that we are bombarded with on a daily basis (most, a flat out rip-off) with tricky ads worked, our society would be slim and trim and without a weight problem. Furthermore, any ad that promises fast, easy, overnight results should be avoided (these ads, fads, and snake oil sales persons in my opinion are just taking your money, so smarten up and get with the program). The only thing that is fast and easy is gaining weight. It is just the way it works and the sooner you realize this the better off you will be and the better off our nation as a whole will be.

The fact is, our society is so overweight it is of national concern. Not only adults, not it is also our children. When people travel to the U. S. from other countries they are shocked at how fat we are. You think they would notice other things but they don't. The biggest thing foreigners notice about us is how fat we are!!! That is something to think about..........

[Throughout the course you may see some points being made twice and it is by design. I want to keep penetrating your way of thinking about food and weight loss and some points need to be made a few times so you get it, so the lights come on and you say ahhhhhhhhhhhhh, this makes sense to me now. Some points just need to be driven home a few times so they stick in your mind. Furthermore, I want you to read this course thoroughly and slowly, and then I want you to reread it a second time or even a third time so you fully grasp all the information (trust me here). Beyond that, I am going to recommend that you keep this information in a filing cabinet or in your library for future reference, too. As the years pass our bodies change, as we get older we tend to slow down and our bodies don't burn the calories like they used to and what worked 10 years ago might not be working today, or if you have a major change in your lifestyle or career or you relocate, things may need fine tuning in your diet. Keep the course somewhere so you can reference it 5 or 10 years from now and if you catch yourself slipping, you can get right back on track by reading the course again and making adjustments.]

I want to get a few things straight right now before you read one more word. As I stated earlier, I am not a doctor or an expert in nutrition!!! This work is my opinion. Consult with your doctor before you do anything we talk about. Let him read the material if you like, and if he sees anything that might jeopardize your health and well-being or if you have a medical condition and he feels there is not hope for you, return the material for a full refund. If your health is already bad and the doctor feels these slight changes will put your life at risk, I really feel sorry for you. But I refuse to put myself in any unnecessary form of liability!!!

Contents

#1 WHAT TO DO IMMEDIATELY 1

#2 SETTING YOUR GOALS 3

#2A GOALS / WEIGHT LOSS CALCULATOR 7

#3 LOOKING AT FOOD DIFFERENTLY 11

#4 CHANGING YOUR EATING HABITS 13

#5 TAKING YOUR MIND OFF FOOD........................... 17

#6 DISCOVER NEW ACTIVITIES TO BURN CALORIES19

#6A MORE ON ACTIVITIES AND THE CALORIES
BURNED 23

#7 HOW TO AVOID THE CONVENIENT STORE
SNACKS THAT = THE CONVENIENT EXTRA UN-
WANTED POUNDS 25

#8 WHY YOU MUST SHOP DIFFERENTLY FROM THIS
DAY FORWARD WHEN YOU GO GROCERY SHOP-
PING 29

#8A COOK, COOK, COOK..................................... 32

#8B THE FINANCIAL SIDE.................................... 34

#9 HOW TO EASILY MAINTAIN YOUR WEIGHT
THROUGHOUT THE HOLIDAYS INSTEAD OF
GAINING 5 OR 10 POUNDS 36

#10 HOW TO AVOID EATING TOO MUCH WHEN YOU
GO OUT FOR DINNER AND WHY YOU MUST STOP
OR CUT WAY BACK ON GOING TO THE ALL YOU
CAN EAT BUFFET 39

#10A THE ALL YOU CAN EAT BUFFET.................. 43

#11 HOW TO HANDLE THE UNEXPECTED LUNCH OR
DINNER DATE WHEN YOU'RE NOT HUNGRY 45

#12   UNDERSTANDING CALORIES AND FOOD............ 47

#13   WHY MOST PEOPLE CAN'T EAT 3 BIG MEALS
       PER DAY AND WHY YOU CAN'T SNACK BETWEEN
       MEALS, WHILE DRIVING, WHEN WATCHING TV,
       OR LATE AT NIGHT JUST BEFORE NIGHTNIGHT 50

#14   POISON VS. FOOD 53

#15   LOSING THE SCALE AND THE DISAPPOINT-
       MENT 57

#16   GETTING TO THE ROOT OF THE PROBLEM 60

#17   ABOUT 300 MILLION PEOPLE IN THE U. S. AND
       ABOUT 6 BILLION ON PLANET EARTH.................. 62

#18   EATING THE FOODS YOU LOVE 65

#19   SERVING SIZES, THEN AND NOW 69

#20   READING LABELS FOR CALORIES AND INGREDI-
       ENTS 73

#21   THINKING ABOUT THE CHILDREN 75

#22   BREAKING THE CYCLE.................................... 79

#23   A CHAT WITH MY BROTHER.................................. 80

#24   YOU DIDN'T GET FAT OVERNIGHT AND YOU'RE
       NOT GOING TO GET SLIM OVERNIGHT................. 82

#25   ADJUSTING FOR A LIFETIME OF SUCCESS.......... 85

#26   TAKE A GOOD LOOK AROUND AT SOCIETY....... 88

#27   TAKING ACTION.. 93

#28   LOW STANDARDS 95

#29   CHANGING YOUR IDENTITY................................. 100

#1 WHAT TO DO IMMEDIATELY

The very first thing you need to do over the next couple of weeks and up to one month is think about your eating habits. You need to think about exactly what you eat every day and when and where you eat. You need to look at how many times you go out for dinner (are you going out for dinner because you are bored?), how many times you go out for lunch, how many meals a day you eat during the week, and how your eating habits change on the weekend. When you stop for gas, are you buying junk food, soda, sweets? Are you snacking between meals, are you snacking at work, are you snacking while you drive, are you snacking while you watch TV? You need to know exactly everything you eat and drink!!! I recommend doing this over a 2 to 4 week period so you get the best cross section of your eating habits. I don't feel it is necessary to write everything down that you eat and drink but you can if you want (most people are very lazy and want everything done for them and won't stick to writing everything down everyday). I feel it is best to keep mental notes, once you start paying attention to your eating habits you will see patterns and you will also see plenty of room for improvement and plenty of opportunities to control your abuse of food intake (if you will just stop and think about it before you shove it into your mouth like there is no tomorrow) and never starve yourself again or deprive yourself of foods you love and never ride the diet/ weight loss roller coaster again. Personally, I never write anything down, it is just not convenient enough for me and for most people with a busy schedule.

I make mental notes. Then you never have to look for your notes and there is no excuse that you didn't write something down and you give up because your notes are not complete and you can't remember what you are suppose to be doing. Furthermore, mental notes keep your mind sharp.

However, <u>if you like writing things down</u> and keeping track of every calorie you eat, I highly recommend you make a simple 7 day chart and track all your meals and add up all the calories that you eat per day and see if this chart opens your eyes and shows you why you have a weight problem. Look, this is not rocket science. Once you know how many calories you need on a daily basis and multiply this number x 7 days in a week you will have a very accurate number of calories needed to maintain your current weight. When you add up the calories that you ate over the course of the week and subtract the number of calories you actually need to maintain your current weight you will see why you are gaining weight. I think this simple chart will be an eye opener for most people. The bottom line here is (regardless if you use the chart or mental notes) do what works for you. <u>But remember, if you are ever going to win the battle of the bulge, you must know these numbers!!!</u>

Over this observation period I want you to monitor your weight and also how your clothes fit. I really don't want you to lose weight in the first 2 to 4 weeks. I just want you to monitor your eating habits, monitor your weight, monitor how your clothes feel and monitor how you feel about yourself and your eating habits, all the time thinking about areas where you can improve and start adjusting your poor diet habits and in return adjust your weight forever. After you feel you have a really good idea of your eating habits you can move on to the next step.

#2 SETTING YOUR GOALS

Each person must decide exactly what they want to accomplish with their diet. You must ask yourself exactly what do you want to do? Do you want to drop 1 dress size or do you need to drop 4? Do you want to lose 10 pounds or do you need to drop 50? Do you just want to maintain your current size for the rest of your life and not have to worry about the pounds adding on? Has your doctor ordered you to slim down or else!? You must know exactly what you want to achieve before you start!!! This next line is one of the most important things I will tell you and you must understand this, regardless of the false promises that you have been told about the miracle juices or the magic pills or the exercise equipment.

OK, here it is.............. You didn't gain the weight overnight and you are not going to lose it overnight.

As far as I am concerned there is no quick fix and my proof is, with all the so called quick fix products that are on the market and a society that is still overweight and doesn't seem to have a clue. People are spending billions of dollars every year looking for the overnight miracle cure and wind up being disappointed with their short term results and most even wind up gaining weight because they get depressed because they failed again. You need to get beyond the quick fix thinking. You need to realize there is no quick fix, or everyone would be slim, trim, and happy about their weight. I say it again because it is so important. You didn't gain the weight overnight and you are not going to lose it overnight!!! Furthermore, once you understand my way of thinking about weight loss you will be able to maintain a healthy weight throughout your life.

Let me ask you a few very important questions. When you cross a busy intersection do you look most of the time, some of the time or all of the time? Think about it. Well, chances are you are still alive and reading this material because you always look both ways every time and triple check before you cross. If you only check occasionally or when you feel like it for speeding traffic it is only a matter of time before you get splattered by a bus!!! Do you drive your car safely with your eyes open every second you are behind the wheel, or do you close your eyes here and there or sleep at the wheel and take a chance on killing yourself? Do you brush your teeth occasionally and hope for the best, or do you brush your teeth thoroughly AM and PM every day? Most people brush their teeth at least twice a day because they know if they don't the consequences might be disastrous. What I don't understand is why people don't think about eating the same way as they do when they think about brushing their teeth, driving their car or crossing a busy street. My point here is you must think about what you eat very carefully everyday for the rest of your life. If you don't and you become obese and your heart explodes or you kidneys fail and you drop dead prematurely it is not going to do you much good to have nice healthy teeth in your dead body. Just something to think about.......... The above analogies are exactly how you must eat from here on out if you want to lose weight and maintain a healthy weight over the long haul. You must start thinking about everything you put into your mouth every time you eat, not just sometime or most of the time, but every time you eat or drink anything!!! The sooner you accept this as fact and deal with it in your mind, the sooner you will be on to adjusting your weight forever and never be burdened again by a weight problem. I am not saying to have flip charts and a notebook for reference every time you are eating or drinking something, but I am saying you need to have mental notes and think about some things. Am I hungry or am I just eating because it is lunch time? Am I hungry or am I going out to dinner because I am bored? Am I hungry or am I eating these chips and soda because they taste good? You must start thinking about everything that you eat and I mean everything, everyday, for the rest of your life!!!

Each person must set their own realistic goal and check with their doctor, then they must take action. I highly recommend you write your goals down and you also write down your approach that you will take to achieve your goal. A goal that is not written down is just a thought and it is not (thought alone) very powerful. A goal written down is very powerful, a plan of attack is even more powerful. Be very specific and set dates for achieving your goal. It is said that about only 5 to 10% of the population have written goals, things they want to achieve in life, and the 5 to 10% with written goals have a net worth equal to the 90% with no plan, no goals.

I heard that little bit of information about setting goals a few years ago and I thought it was rather interesting. I remember chatting with a friend right after the new year and we were not very happy with our lives and what we had accomplished and we were basically sitting around having a bitch session. It was a Sunday. Monday morning I went into work and did nothing all day except think about what I wanted to accomplish and where I wanted to be in the future. I thought and wrote all day long. At the end of the day I created an exact road map for the rest of my life. I had filled 10 sheets of paper with goals/dreams that I wanted to achieve this year, short term and long term - a dream house I wanted to live in, a lake house I wanted to build to relax and enjoy life, the cars I wanted to drive, and the lifestyle that I wanted. I wrote my goals down with very specific details and time frames in which I wanted to accomplish them. I basically designed a road map for my life that would take me anywhere I wanted to go. It was one of the most powerful things I have ever done in my life and it changed my life forever!!! It has been a couple of years since I wrote down my goals and as I review them (sometimes on a daily basis) I am very pleased with what I have accomplished already. I highly recommend you do this exercise. Get a notebook and a pen and sit down for an afternoon or an entire day as I did and write down your goals/dreams in great detail.

<u>Take action and do this exercise!!!</u> If you want to lose weight, build a dream house, drive a dream car, find a great life mate, get a better job, improve your marriage, take a dream vacation, or have

better relationships with your children. Take some time and write your goals down. <u>With consistent action in the right direction</u> I believe 99% of the population can reach and maintain a healthy weight. <u>With consistent action in the right direction you can achieve much greatness in many areas of your life.</u>

#2A GOALS / WEIGHT LOSS CALCULATOR

Once you have a realistic goal in mind this section will give you some idea as to how long it will take to reach your goal. Let's start out with some basics. We know for sure that there are seven days in a week and fifty two weeks in a year. We also know that there are about 3500 calories in a pound. So if you want to lose 10 pounds that is about 35,000 calories (20 pounds is about 70,000 calories). Now, are there ten thousand ways to lose the weight, or two? If you watch a lot of TV you might think there are ten thousand products for you to buy. Think about it for a minute. This is a serious question!!! Lucky for you, common sense says that there are only two basic ways to lose the 10 pounds/35,000 calories. One, eat 35,000 less calories over a period of time. Two, burn 35,000 extra calories over a period of time. Now, let's do some thinking together, some simple math and get to the root of the problem. Now, after doing the first exercise in chapter one of monitoring our diet habits we need to see where we can start to save calories, especially the poison calories that we will discuss in section #14 [poison vs. food] each person will be able to see where they can start to shave calories on a consistent basis to slowly but surely (remember there are no quick fixes) win the war on being overweight. Now let's look at some examples. If you want to lose the 10 pounds over the course of one year you will have to shave only 100 calories per day from your diet and not change anything else and simple math tells us that you will lose 10 pounds in one year. 100 calories x 7 days = 700 calories per week x 52 weeks in a year = 36,400 calories. Now, if every man, woman and child in the U. S. can't cut 100 calories from their diet every single day and not even miss them I would be very surprised!!! This is what I call getting to the root of the problem, breaking it down in simple terms, doing simple math and making small changes over a period of time that will have a positive affect on your weight and hopefully your overall health and well- being.

In the first month when you were thinking about your eating habits and the food that you consume I hope you were seeing plenty of opportunity to shave unnecessary calories from your diet and never even miss one of them. Another reason this course works is because it is per individual, it is based on exactly what you would normally be doing on a daily basis and just shaving a few calories here and there. Now you may be saying a year is a long time to lose 10 pounds and to a point I agree, but bottom line, it must work if you stick with it, unless you have a serious medical condition it will work!!! Moreover, it's better than gaining another 10 pounds and heading for obesity!!! Even if you went the entire year making small lifestyle changes and maintained your current weight and got your eating under control and didn't gain an ounce, I must say again, it's better than gaining. I have seen people on diets their whole lives, I have seen people try every diet on the market, I have seen people try every pill that was advertised on TV and I have seen people try exercise with very disappointing results. Furthermore, all they seemed to do was whine about their problem, I am on this diet today, that diet tomorrow, starving myself today, pig out tomorrow, I can't eat bread for a month or any donuts, or everything I eat is fat free no taste artificial yuck, blahblahblah. Yet they are so excited that they will lose 20 pounds in a month and their weight problem will be solved forever. Sad to say they have unrealistic goals and have been sold a bill of goods that in most cases will fail. Have you ever seen this person or has this ever been you? The worst part is they always seem miserable, they always seem to be depriving themselves of foods they love and they never seem to get ahead on the weight loss!!! OK, we all have been there and done that. Let's get back to the 10 pounds, one year and 100 calories per day. The main reason I started there is because I wanted everyone to be able to achieve the goal. Even if it took 3 years to achieve a 30 pound loss and it was permanent, and a slow, healthy change and the <u>new healthy eating/lifestyle and the new habits/changes lasted a lifetime,</u> in my opinion it is very much worth it. How long have you been on different diets up to this point? Something else you might want to think about is if you don't get with the program and start paying attention and lowering your calorie intake, and 3 years pass, and now you have gained 30 or 50 pounds, heading for obesity or overworking your heart until it explodes out of your chest, or over loading your knees until they fail. My goal is not to shock you here, but I do want to get your attention. I do want you to think about what you are doing to your body and to your quality of life by over eating.

OK, lets look a little deeper and see how some can speed this process up. Again we will use the 10 pound example. If you can shave 200 calories per day on a consistent basis and again I believe most people can achieve this without any problem, you will be cutting the time in half. 200 calories a day x 7 days = 1400 calories per week x 26 weeks = 36,400 calories. I feel this is a realistic number that most people can comfortably achieve without much problem. Now, let's take things one step further and add burning some extra calories to the formula (remember, we said there are only 2 basic ways to lose weight - eat less calories and burn more calories). If the average person can add burning only 200 extra calories (walking for 1 hour) per day to the formula (we will go into detail in section #6 about new ways to burn calories), which I feel is very possible for most healthy people, you can shave the 10 pounds off in 13 weeks, again cutting the time in half. Now this = losing 10 pounds in basically 3 months, 20 pounds in 6 months, 30 pounds in 9 months and 40 pounds in a year, by just making some minor adjustments to your lifestyle, never starving yourself, never over exerting yourself, basically paying attention to what and when you eat and <u>thinking yourself thin,</u> trim and healthy. This may be a little aggressive for some people, but the main thing I wanted to show everyone is that it is possible to slim down and lose a lot of unwanted weight in one year and change your life for the better. Even if you took a steady conservative approach of eating 100 calories less everyday and burning 100 calories more everyday, you would drop about 20 pounds by the end of the year. A combination of 200 calories either burned or not consumed x 7 days per week x 52 weeks = 20 pounds lost in one year. Simple math: 200 x 7 = 1400 calories x 52 weeks = 72,800 calories saved for the year, divided by 3500 calories in a pound = a 20 pound loss. 100 calories saved per day x 7 days per week x 52 weeks per year = a 10 pound loss. 100 x 7 = 700 x 52 = 36,400 divide by 3500 = 10.40 LBS. lost. In a nutshell, you can figure every unit of 100 calories (either burned or not consumed) saved per day for one year will equal a 10 LB weight loss. These savings must be everyday!!!

I really feel most people don't have a grip on just how delicate of a balancing act it is between maintaining a healthy weight and being obese. Saving or burning 700 extra calories a week is not a big deal, and when done every week you will lose weight. It has to work without fail unless you have something severely wrong with you. The eye opener here is if your entire week is perfect and you binge on 1 extra chocolate chip muffin and 1 regular 12 ounce soda at the convenient mart you have blown the whole week. As you start getting a feel for just how many calories are in our favorite treats and foods we eat everyday you will understand how the whole week can be blown on 3 jelly donuts.

#3 LOOKING AT FOOD DIFFERENTLY

In this section I want you to identify your problem areas. We all have them and they are different for everyone. But we all must identify where we are losing the battle. Do you snack between meals, do you snack while watching TV, do you snack late at night, do you snack at work or while driving, do you eat too many meals a day, do you pig out on weekends, do you eat too much per meal, do you power lunch during the week at work, do you eat junk food 24 - 7, do you eat fast food for lunch everyday, are you drowning in a sugar bath of biggie sodas and chocolates? Do you go out for dinner because you are bored, do you eat to socialize, are you a lazy slob? OK, I hope you get the point here. You need to start looking at food a different way. If you can identify one solid problem area in your life and get it handled and never go back to the old ways, you may have won the battle. The great part about my approach is that you have to make little changes over the long term. If you left 6 bites of food on your plate (instead of licking your plate clean or when you know you are stuffed you grab another scoop of this or another slice of that) every meal, everyday, you would probably never have a weight problem. If you can just remember this fact every time you are eating to be a little disciplined, a little more conservative, everyday for the rest of your life, you will be much better off in the long run. Up until the last 50 years or so, people ate to live, now I think people live to eat. It seems like we have nothing left to do in our cushy lives except eat. Instead of looking at food in a healthy way to nourish our bodies and sustain our lives we look at food as a hobby, a sport, a pastime, or something to do when we are bored. We need to start to look at food again from a nourishing point of view. Once we start looking at food differently, we can win the battle over buying and eating junk foods. We can slow the frequency in which we dine out on over processed unhealthy foods. This little change in your thinking will make you think twice before you load your cart at the mega mart with all those flavor enhanced, over salted, over preserved, over sugared prepackaged convenience foods, that have little or no nutritional value and do nothing for our bodies except make us obese and give us heart disease. <u>We need to start to look at food from a nutritious point of view again, the sooner the better.</u>

#4 CHANGING YOUR EATING HABITS

Recently we have heard about the Europeans being so much more healthy and fit than the U. S. and we have pinned all their success on red wine. So here in the states the sales of red wine have sky rocketed I guess. Then we hear how much cream, butter, chocolate, meat, cheese and other rich, tasty foods they are consuming with ostensibly no ill side effects. Did you ever wonder what they seem to be doing right and what we are obviously doing wrong? I would say red wine is good but I am not so sure it is the panacea we have been dreaming of. I do believe, though, that we need to take some lessons from the Europeans here.

Without a doubt I love to cook and I love to eat, but it seems in the U. S. that eating is a sport or a hobby, he who consumes the most wins. Furthermore, we seem to eat with speed so we can get on to the next task in our lives. I really think most people eat until their stomach simply will not hold anymore food or drink, then we stop eating. Even while dining out it seems to be a fast paced marathon. Order as quick as possible, pig out on the free bread, then the monster appetizers, then the main course and as long as we are so wealthy (and fat and happy) why not order a dessert and split it? All the while this whole scene is moving at such a fast pace almost to see how fast we can get in and get out and the restaurant can fill that table again with fat, hungry customers.

The essence here is that we need to slow down when we eat, we need to taste/enjoy our food instead of inhaling it. If you watch European movies or cooking shows or shows on their culture/lifestyles you will see the Europeans are passionate about their food and meal times. I observe them eating slowly and savoring every bite, I observe them enjoying the meal and usually the good company and conversation of friends and family. I see them enjoying rich foods made with cream and butter (especially the French). I see them enjoying full meals of meat and fish and vegetables, I see them enjoying dessert. What I didn't see was snacking between meals, and little or no junk food lying around and they did not consume huge Americana size monster portions. Another thing I think may be making a difference is their pace. Slowing down gives your stomach time to signal the brain that it is full and no more eating is necessary.

I have tested myself to see just how smart my body was and I was amazed with my results. Everyone should be able to try this simple test. This is what I did when I got home from work one night when I was starving after a long day. (Ever heard the line about my eyes being bigger than my belly? I think many of us suffer from this problem.) As I said I was starving, so I made a huge pile of food because my brain said huge quantity, we are starving here dude. So I made a huge plate and sat down to eat, but I ate with a plan, and thought about some things like slowing the pace of consumption and actually tasting the food and enjoying every bite instead of inhaling it. I sipped my beverage instead of guzzling it like a camel heading for the Mojave, I flipped through a new magazine I picked up on the way home and skimmed through an article of interest, and I played some music at low volume to slow the pace and ease the tension of the day. Now here is what I discovered personally - after about 15 to 20 minutes of enjoying my food, sipping my beverage and skimming through my magazine, I noticed I had only consumed about half of what my brain and my eyes thought I should eat that evening. More important, my stomach was signaling my brain that it was reaching the full mark and my eating further slowed. Furthermore, this delicious food that I prepared was not so appealing towards the end as I became comfortably full. Roughly only 20 minutes had passed and I was not starving anymore, a few more minutes passed and I pushed away my plate that was only half eaten. Now, this is not willpower!!! This is how smart your body is if you just let it function properly and let it do its job. I fully believe if my pace was rapid I could have easily consumed the huge plate that I prepared, stuffing it all down in 10 to 15 minutes and walking away feeling like a stuffed pig. If you are constantly walking away from meals feeling like a stuffed pig I believe you are eating too much too fast.

I think everyone should do this simple test or something similar and see what your time frame is for your brain to get the full signal from your stomach. See how much time passes when you sit down to eat, from start to finish, and I think you might be surprised how fast we eat in this country. The amazing thing about the brain getting the full signal is, I could have had my most favorite meal prepared by a 5 star chef placed in front of me at this time and I would not be interested in eating anymore because I was simply full. If you just think about this it will make sense. <u>Again, this is not willpower, this is your body being brilliant.</u> Willpower is why we are all obese, willpower is not powerful enough to keep us away from the German chocolate cake when we know we are already full to the point of bursting out of our clothes!!!

[tangent] Have you ever heard the saying you are either a cook or a baker? For the most part it is a true statement. As I have told you many times I love to cook and I love to eat. I am a great cook and I like to bake and I usually bake well but it could be better. I was reading a book on baking world class pastry and breads and one thing I read changed everything, one simple line that made sense to me and stuck. <u>Baking is in the details.</u> After reading those five words it completely changed my thinking. Ahhhhhhhhhh, I thought, baking is in the details. That is the secret of great bakers, they are very detail oriented, they are very precise. When most people cook and me included, we cook by feel and most times on dishes that are prepared frequently it's without a recipe and without precision, a pinch of this a pinch of that, a handful of this and a bunch of that, cooking times can vary, weights can vary and measurements can be very arbitrary, as the dish nears completion we adjust the seasonings to taste before serving and whaala, good eats!!! Before I read those 5 words (baking is in the details), I used to bake as I cooked, not realizing that I had to be very precise when I was baking to get the desired results. Now when I bake, I shift gears and change my mindset to the precise

mode. For those who cook and bake I hope you are thinking deeply about this. Personally, I will never bake the same ever again. Now I know the secret of great world class bakers. Now I consider myself a great cook and a great baker.

I hope something in this course sticks and you say ahhhhhhhhhh, there is the secret I have been looking for, or this makes sense and I can do this. Just like my baking discovery (5 words) that changed my life from being a great cook to being a great cook and great baker..............

#5 TAKING YOUR MIND OFF FOOD

I want to open this chapter with one question that I want you to think about. Do you eat because you are hungry or because you are bored? I really feel most people eat the extra unnecessary calories out of boredom, I see very few people passing out because they are starving. Think about something.............. did you know a person 100 pounds overweight can go an entire year eating only every other day and just get back to their regular weight? So I doubt you will pass out from starvation not having your snack between breakfast and lunch. I see way too many people snacking between meals and even on the job in professional positions and usually they are fatties!!!

First off I think it is very unprofessional snacking on the job. Second, it is totally unnecessary and totally undisciplined!!! It kills me to see a person struggling with their weight on the verge of being obese and they are snacking on low fat foods and diet soda on the job. You are working fer Christ sake!!! Focus on your job and stop thinking about food. I don't care if it is low cal/no cal, in my opinion you need to stop shoveling food in your face. Your body does not know what to do with this poison except store it on your belly and your ass, and when it runs out of room there it starts storing fat on every inch of your body. If your body could talk it would say why are you pouring all this poison into me that I have no need for? Your body can't talk so it responds to your negative actions by making you fat. [point] If the only thing on your mind is food, you are screwed!!!

Every person must answer this question and be honest with yourself. Do you constantly think about food? <u>If all you can think about is food, you must start getting something else on your mind</u> and this will be different for everyone. Focus on your job, focus on a hobby, focus on positive thoughts, focus on your relationship, focus on your kids, focus on your finances, focus on being a disciplined person, get your mind off of food. If you are eating because you are bored you must start getting this under control immediately!!! Every single calorie consumed because you are bored is a poison calorie that your body does not need!!! I hope you get this and it sinks in. Start doing something constructive. Try picking up a book and reading instead of picking up a snack. Be creative here and <u>take action and make positive changes.</u> As long as I am waxing taking action and making changes, I want to make another important point. Why on earth would an intelligent person keep doing the same thing over and over and over and over again without getting the desired results/ change and keep going down that same road? If you have been on different diets for the last 10 years and you are still overweight, when will you stop the madness, when will you change your approach? <u>How stupid do you have to be to keep doing something that isn't working?</u> Do you need to be slapped across your face to be brought to your senses? My point, if what you are doing isn't working, change what you are doing, change your approach, change your way of thinking, change your habits, change the tools you are using, change your methods, until you get your desired result, <u>stop going down the wrong road that is not taking you where you want to go.</u> You can apply this new way of thinking in many areas of your life!!!

#6 DISCOVER NEW ACTIVITIES TO BURN CALORIES

Now as discussed in section 2A, we are going to look deeper into this and discover new ways to burn the calories away and also become <u>more active</u> and get our bodies moving. Personally I believe most of the overweight problem and poor health can be pinned to the fact that most people are very lazy and most people are very inactive. Think about this - in the 1940's and 50's I think very few people had any problem with maintaining a healthy weight. My proof is if you view old movies or see pictures from that era most people were very slim. People ate healthy and hearty meals, most people ate 3 times a day and still they were very slim. Hardly without any concern about meat or bread or dessert. I think one of the main reasons is the fact that in that era people were very active, men worked hard in construction, farming and manufacturing and were burning major calories as they worked hard on a daily basis. Women for the most part stayed home to raise the children and keep the home and did not have all the modern day conveniences of today, so in turn worked very hard to keep the house up and also cooking the meals.

My point here is people were very active and worked very hard on a daily basis and usually seven days a week. Health clubs and fitness equipment were not of much use because when people got home from work or through with their day they were exhausted from their daily hard labor and they were burning enough calories where obesity was not much of an issue. In the 60's and 70's we started to see a shift in jobs and also in modern conveniences for the home to make life more easy. We also started seeing things like the TV dinner and a flood of prepackaged and processed foods to fit with the more fast paced society that we were becoming. More and more people left the country and headed for the city and the office job and I think the changes started to affect the way people lived and our lifestyles forever. I really feel that in the 60's and 70's things started changing for the worse, although people were still pretty slim and healthy I feel the change started. Through the 80's and 90's we went fully from a manufacturing/construction booming/farming country to consumers and to a country who imports most of its consumables. Now we are into the 21st century and feeling all the ill effects of our modern society and all the ill effects of all the modern conveniences that everyone is dependent on and all the ill effects of having everything done for us by a machine or appliance or a computer.

In my opinion we have become a very inactive and lazy society. We have become a society that sits on our ass at work and then goes home and sits some more in front of a TV or computer because there is nothing to do because everything is being done for us. Think about something - who actually works for 10 hours a day doing hard manual labor? We have machines to do that for us now. Even most manufacturing jobs are so automated or robotic that most people again are sitting around watching the computer screen or sit there and press a few buttons and make sure the thing doesn't blow up or stop running.

My point is we are not a very active society and it is now taking its toll on our health and well-being and causing weight issues with the masses. Perhaps we have taken a round about way to discovering new ways to get active and burn calories but I wanted to drive the point home about the shift in the work place and the fact that most people do very little at their job anymore and that we have become consumers and pencil pushers. The more we sit on our butts the heavier our society will become. Something to think about...............

You hear all these people saying you should get a nice 20 minute workout per day to keep your heart healthy, think about people 50 years ago that worked hard all day long for 8 or 10 hours and didn't stop for 4 coffee breaks. Even at a conservative 7 total hours worked x 60 minutes, that is a whopping 420 minute daily workout. That's probably why there wasn't much heart disease back then and if you were obese chances are you had a severe medical condition. To take this little story one step further, if we do a simple calculation and figure they were doing a good days labor for a good days pay and burning maybe 250 to 300 calories per hour (and some were burning a lot more!!!) x 7 hours that = about 2000 calories they were burning at work alone, <u>more than most of us burn in 24 hours today.</u> Let's play with these numbers here for a bit. If a hard working man was burning 2000 calories at work (8 hours), 800 calories while sitting around the house, (and you know darn well men weren't sitting around much 50 years ago) driving or watching TV (8 hours), and 400 calories while sleeping (8 hours), that easily totals to about 3000 calories a day he could consume and still stay very slim and healthy. That is 3 hearty meals (actually cooked) of 1000 calories each. Fast forward 50 years, we still want to eat 3 meals a day like the good old days, but we are simply not burning the calories.

I hope you can see how we must change our thinking/eating to adjust to our new 21st century lifestyles. I hope you can understand why we are wrestling with obesity and poor health on such a large scale. I hope you can see why most of us can't eat 3 big meals a day. I hope you start getting a clue here why we are such an overweight nation.

Personally I have a desk job and consider myself a pencil pusher. I also hate working out and probably will never join a gym. As I said earlier I am just an ordinary person like you. As I got older I realized that I must discover some activities that I enjoyed to keep active and maintain my weight and get my butt off the couch and get active. Again, I am like most ordinary people, I hate working out, I hate counting calories and I hate not being comfortable in my clothes. The bottom line, the key to staying active is find some things that you love to do and stick with them. Everyone must find activities that interest them and are not a drag or a pain.

As we said there are not ten thousand ways to adjust your weight, in my opinion there are only two. Eat less or burn more calories. Most people are so narrow minded and such <u>suckers</u> for tricky ads for exercise equipment they wind up buying the equipment, stick with it for a few months and they hate every minute of it and it winds up in the garage or basement or sold at a garage sale for pennies on the dollar. Or you buy a membership to a health club with the best intentions and go a few times and say the heck with that. It's a fact that a lot of people have health club memberships but a large percentage stop going after a few months and don't renew. Again if you hate doing it you are not going to stick with it. This is very important!!! If you bought a treadmill and hated that, then you bought a stationary bike and hated that, and then you bought the next guaranteed contraption and that didn't work so you bought weights and again you didn't stick with it because you hated it. You must change the way you think!!! If it is not working you must change what you are doing, instead of doing the same thing over and over and over. Wake up!!! And change what isn't working to something that will. <u>Don't keep making the same mistake over and over and over.</u> Change what you are doing.............. This applies not only to weight management but you can use this in all areas of your life.

I hope you are getting the point here. You must get active and get your butt moving. It must be an enjoyable activity that you can stick with. I will share a few of the things that I replaced the failed exercise equipment with that got me active and off the couch and moving. Personally, I love being outdoors. So instead of focusing on things I couldn't do or hated doing, I focused on things I could do and you need to do the same. I don't want to hear you whining I can't do that or I can't afford that or I am too old or blahblahblah. <u>Focus on what you can do, ask yourself, what can I do!?</u> I own land in the country and loved spending time there. It is 60 acres and mostly woods. I absolutely love going there and walking the trails that I cut myself and clearing brush and cutting wood. It is the best exercise and the best form of relaxation for me. I love it!!! I don't have to force myself to go there and work, I look forward to going and can't wait to get there to work hard and burn calories. I also love to walk, it is not a huge burn of calories but it still gets you moving and it is much better than sitting on the couch shoving junk food in your mouth. <u>Discover something you love doing and stick with it.</u> I hate excuses, I love solutions!!! Find something you love doing and stick with it!!!

#6A MORE ON ACTIVITIES AND THE CALORIES BURNED

The point I want to make in this section and I admit I didn't have a clue either (until I did some research) was how much you had to do to burn off calories. Furthermore, I hope you will now understand how you can look at a big steak or a piece of cake and see the pounds pack on. Most people think as I did, I can eat like a pig and if I walk for an hour it will burn right off. Wrong!!!

It seems like you eat a little extra and it packs right on as extra weight and for the most part it Is true. Think about your body and comfortable weight like a glass that is filled to the very top with water (do a visual here folks). If you add just a tiny bit more water the glass overflows. It is the same with our bodies. I feel so many are like the full glass, just bordering on spilling over and gaining more weight and the slightest bit of extra food consumed starts adding on to our weight or basically spilling over like the full glass of water and our body catches the overflow, the little bit of extra food consumed and stores it on our bodies and the scale creeps higher and higher over time, ounce by ounce, drop by drop. If I designed our bodies, I would have designed us opposite, eat like a pig, walk for 10 minutes and lose weight. Well, that is a pipe dream. Let's get back to the real world.

I am now going to give you a small sample of activities and the calories burned. I am using general and conservative figures here for examples only. I want to open your eyes here and show you how few calories we burn in our daily cushy lives. If you want more accurate figures you can go online and I recommend you do this. [If you are serious about getting your weight problem handled it is almost a must that you go online and see exactly what your body type needs for calories daily, the reason for me saying it is a must do is because I have been talking with a lot of people about my course and when I ask them to give me a ball park figure on how many calories they thought they were burning in a normal day, they either didn't have a clue or they were not even close!!! If you ever want to get your weight problem handled you must know this figure and it must be accurate.] There are websites where you can enter your gender, weight, height, age, and it will show you what your body type burns per hour doing a wide variety of activities. Again, these are approximate numbers here for a 150 pound man too give you an idea of the calories burned in one hour of activity. Sleeping, 50. Watching TV, 100. Housework, walking, 150. Mowing the lawn (riding) 200. Riding a bike 5 mph, raking leaves, golfing (power cart) 250. Gardening, badminton, bowling, light swimming, 350. Going upstairs, singles tennis, jogging, downhill skiing, basketball, 500. Running, fast swimming, cross country skiing, rowing machine, 800. Again, these are estimates. I highly recommend you go online and get your exact figures for your body type and size. My numbers are to give you an idea only and help show you why you can't think you can pig out, then go walk for an hour and solve all your weight problems. Before I looked up my chart online, I thought I burned about 500 calories an hour walking!!! Wow, was I wrong. Even with my sample chart you can see how strenuous the activity is before you even dream of hitting the 500 calories burned per hour activity. It opened my eyes and I hope it opens yours too. Furthermore, it helped me come to grips with the facts why most people are having weight problems and why we have to change our way of thinking.

#7 HOW TO AVOID THE CONVENIENT STORE SNACKS THAT = THE CONVENIENT EXTRA UNWANTED POUNDS

When I was growing up about 20 years ago I remember gassing my truck up to go to high school for my senior year. I remember gas was hitting an all time high of one dollar per gallon (this was 1981). But I also remember the gas station too, and this is my point to the story. I lived in a rural area and convenient marts were not even dreamed of in my area. We had a couple of small gas stations that sold gas and one was full service so you never got out of your vehicle. They filled your car with gas, you paid, and you took off. Both gas stations in my town did have a small store with an old display case that had a few old chocolate bars, some chewing gum, a small rack with some smokes, and a cooler with some soda in it. Bottom line, you went to gas up your vehicle, not buy junk food and get lunch.

Now, fast forward 20 years. The old gas stations I used to go to are closed up and they have been replaced with a mega convenient mart anchored with gas pumps. It seems some brilliant gas station owner figured out that most every person on earth has to fill their car with gas once or twice a week. He also figured out that he was losing a ton of profit by letting these frequent customers get away with buying only gas or gas and a 50 cent soda or 25 cent pack of gun. I can only imagine it was one greedy/creative/brilliant shop owner that brought about the whole concept of the mega convenient mart anchored with the gas pumps. Once they saw that the new model worked it was only a matter of I would guess 20 years that every town of decent size has one or even three convenient marts. Now, for the shop owners, this is a real money maker, same customer, except instead of generating a gas sale only, he is generating mega profit per customer per stop because of the add on food/drink sale. (are you starting to get the picture here folks???????).

Don't get me wrong here folks, from a convenience point of view and a business/profit point of view these convenient marts are gold mines. The downside is when you stop for gas how many unnecessary calories of junk food are you buying and packing on your body? Just notice how the stores are laid out!!! All the tempting junk food front and center, the drinks at the back so you have to pass all the other poison foods. Think about this, is their anything of high nutritional value in these convenient marts? I don't think so!!! OK, maybe they have a few old bananas, a few shriveled up apples or oranges, but my point here is the majority of the food on the shelf is over preserved poison!!! High in fat, loaded with artificial everything under the sun, huge calories, all corn syrup (the worst) and of no food value for your body. I will give them credit for the good job on packaging and marketing, but it is coming in the form of a huge negative effect on our nation with the unwanted, unnecessary calories and all the other ill effects on our bodies of junk food. I challenge you to do a little observation yourself next time you stop to gas up. Take a good look at the store, the layout, the marketing, the signs, the packaging, find all the delicious, healthy, nutritious, wholesome food that your body needs and make a mental note. Then I want you to take a good look at all the junk food and just give yourself a rough percentage in your head. I bet you will see that the junk food is 95% or more and if you can actually find something healthy it will be less than 5%!!! Take the challenge for the heck of it and see what you think now of the convenient mart anchored with the gas pumps.

While you're at it I want you to take notice of something else. I want you to look at the calories and the ingredients in some of the things you usually grab and eat. Just for the heck of it see how many calories are in that tasty flavor enhanced muffin with the fancy label and a shelf life of a couple weeks or more and read the long list of ingredients/preservatives/food colorings. Gee, I bet your body is just dying for all that good stuff............... not!!! Look, I am no rocket scientist but I do wonder where the hell they get all those ingredients to make a damn 3 ounce muffin. I will tell you I do like to cook and the last time I made bread or muffins it only took a few ingredients, flour, water, yeast, maybe a few blueberries and a little bit of luck and I have good eats. I just hope you take the time to do this exercise and you realize that maybe that tasty muffin, or whatever you're grabbing on the go made with ingredients from out of this world is really not the best thing for your body or your belly.

Something to think about............... one 450 calorie muffin (we are really beating up the poor muffin so substitute anything you buy here on a consistent basis at the convenient mart that your body absolutely does not need or want) per week x 52 weeks = about 6 pounds of unwanted weight gain over the course of one year. So if your exercise program is perfect and your other eating habits are perfect to maintain your weight, just this one slight fault on a consistent basis throughout the year and you porked on a solid 6 pounds!!! Scary, isn't it???

I would almost bet that everyone reading this material buys and eats every week a lot more than 450 unwanted, unneeded calories of bad/junk food while getting gas. Do you? Perhaps it is time you thought about this more seriously. If this is a problem for you I want you to think about these simple solutions. #1 Pay at the pump and boogie, never going into the store to be tempted. [Make sure you immediately put that cash in an envelope and apply to the credit card. I don't want any of you getting in trouble with your credit cards doing this, especially considering how expensive gas is today!!! Or buy a prepaid gas card each month.] #2 Take a stand and show some self control and think to yourself while inside the store, do I want to fall prey to fancy labels and good marketing, do I want to eat all of those nasty preservatives, does my body need a 24 ounce soda loaded with sugar that my body does not know what to do with except store as fat on my belly (how about a nice refreshing 24 ounce bottle of spring water to hydrate your cells and flush your system, something your body will say aaaaaaaaaaaaa to), am I really starving or is this just too convenient, do I want to pack on 6 or 10 extra pounds this year by slipping up here? Do yourself a favor here and use your brain to make a good decision. <u>Take a stand and show some self control!!!</u> Personally, I think about all the red dye or preservatives that you can't even pronounce on the labels of ingredients, all the fat, all the sugar, and tell myself in my head <u>no</u> and walk away, either empty handed or with a bottle of water and the paper. It is my way of taking a stand and I hope you come up with something creative to take a stand too!!!

#8 WHY YOU MUST SHOP DIFFERENTLY FROM THIS DAY FORWARD WHEN YOU GO GROCERY SHOPPING

Quick question. What is the very first step that an alcoholic must do to quit drinking? Get all the booze out of the house. It goes back to willpower and being in control. Very few people have the discipline to stop drinking if the booze are in the house and easy to get to. I feel it is very similar with food. Furthermore, being obese is just as bad as being a drunk but it hasn't earned the proper stigma yet..............

The first step I want you to take here is to take a good look around at the food you have in your house. The refrigerator, the freezer, the kitchen counter, the cupboards, and the pantry. I want you to take a complete inventory of the foods that you are buying. [I feel strongly that our obesity is a sign of wealth in our country. Think about this - most people can go to the grocery store and pretty much buy whatever they want and whatever looks good.] This is also a good time to identify some obvious problem areas (review section 3 for more on this). You must be honest with yourself here because this is a huge necessary step that I feel must be taken to win the war on obesity!!! Especially if you have children that are bulging at the seams!!! This is the time to identify the food vs. the poison, the wholesome, nutritious food vs. the pure junk food, the solid meal foods that your body needs to be healthy vs. the deadly snacks (I see the snackers whimpering here). This one exercise could change your life forever. Now, as I discussed in section #1 the first 2 to 4 weeks are really about observing your current patterns and just identifying areas where there is room for improvement. After you take a hard look at the food you have on hand I hope your eyes are being opened here, I hope you can see why you are losing the battle of the bulge. Moreover, if you go grocery shopping every week I hope you don't replace some items that you know are no good for you and save your money. Now if you want to get serious and take massive action, you can overhaul your entire on-hand food supply and either toss out the poison or donate what you can to a local food bank!!! I bet if most people took one day and laid all the food they have in their house on the counter and kitchen table and took a hard look at it and started reading the labels and calories and all the artificial ingredients that we are pouring into our bodies, most would be shocked into a new way of life. I challenge you to make 2 piles, one with the pure junk food/poison and the other with wholesome and nutritious foods and see which pile is bigger and what changes need to be made immediately when you are grocery shopping. <u>This change needs to be for the rest of your life!!!</u> At minimum this exercise will open your eyes. The action takers would be on their way to the food bank with a large haul and I hope never to purchase this poison again. This section is all about willpower and discipline. Very few have enough self control to win the war. Why not put the odds in your favor and not bring the bad stuff home?

[tangent] We know we have very little self control/discipline, but you know something, people respect people that show any level of self control. Overall I have pretty good discipline in my life and people give me a lot of respect because they know this fact about me and I apply it in many areas of my life and the long term benefit is huge. Relationships, business, finances and the battle of the bulge, a little self control goes a long way and over the long term makes a huge difference.

This is also a time to be creative and change your bad habits. The good news is you can still enjoy some of this stuff on occasion but you cannot have it lying around in quantity 24 - 7 if you ever want to get the upper hand on long term weight control. A box of fresh jelly donuts .... (insert your favorite sweet treat on this line) will overtake my strong will every time and I imagine your favorite junk food will, too. I could easily eat 12 jelly donuts in 2 days all the time knowing this was excessive for me, but I love them!!! Until I started shopping differently and going to the bakery at my grocery store and buying 2 jelly donuts instead of a dozen and only on occasion is how I creatively got power over the almighty jelly donut. Now, when I do get them I savor every bite. I never deprive myself of the food I love, but I have cut back a huge amount on the quantity I consume. Some of the real bad food/poison I have cut out of my life by 100%. Each person must identify their own downfalls and be creative in dealing with either cutting the real bad stuff 100% or cutting way back to tolerable portions that will have your body smiling. We all know the bad stuff is no good for our bodies and it does nothing to make us healthy but we still keep buying it and we keep eating it. Sometimes it just takes a nudge in the right direction, a little wake up call, <u>a good look in the mirror,</u> and most of us intelligent beings can get it handled once and for all. If you make a shopping list before you leave the house you must start making this list differently from this day forward for the rest of your life.

Furthermore, I think that most should establish a budget and go shopping once a week. A budget will limit the spending. A list ensures you get only what is needed and stops you from shopping like you are preparing for a 3 week blizzard, and going weekly you can buy small quantities and fresher foods. Personally, I feel the warehouse clubs with the huge size packaging and bulk packaging were one of the worst ideas ever created and I don't care if you have 12 kids and you think you are saving money. In my opinion it is a wrong way of thinking and buying. <u>I feel strongly, the more we have the more we consume.</u> The larger the container the more we can eat, rather than throw out the product before it expires we pork it down so as not to waste money. All wrong thinking. I can't stress this point enough - we must all shop differently/smarter from this day forward!!!

#8A COOK, COOK, COOK

Personally, I love to cook and I think we have strayed too far away from home cooking. [here we go] Now I know some of you are already whining about having no time. Well boo hoo. I feel most people are very poor managers of their time and if truly you were so busy you should not be fat. If you had so much to do you should not have a weight problem. Soooo busy no time to eat, no time to cook, no time to relax. Poor baby............... [As you will see throughout this course I call it like I see it. I am not into sugar coating, I don't like whiners, I don't like complainers, and I don't like people that don't take responsibility and have to blame everyone else for their ills and never look in the mirror.] I bet if most people sat down and reviewed just how not busy they really are and how bad they manage their time they would be surprised. I heard a statistic that on average Americans watch TV 7 hours per day!!! Not you of course, but the average person in America I bet watches a good 5 to 6 hours per day on a regular basis. Bottom line here is if you are so busy you can't cook then stop snacking between meals and your weight problem will be solved with your high level of daily activity. If you are sitting on your ass watching 5 hours of TV per day, switch to a cooking show and learn how to cook and start cooking real nutritious and delicious food. If you already like to cook and you are a good cook, start cooking more. Discover the fresh food section at your grocery store and actually prepare a real meal. It is time to stop buying the convenient microwaveable foods. It is time to stop buying the bulk of your weekly groceries in the frozen food section.

I saw a TV show on how they made TV dinners and I could not believe how they manipulated the foods. Believe me, you really don't want to know how scientists get a piece of chicken to cook at the same rate as peas and like magic they are done at the same time. I was never a fan of frozen food and after seeing that show on the making of TV dinners I hope you think about avoiding them too. Maybe it is time you asked yourself how do they do that, how do they get a piece of chicken to cook in the same amount of time as peas or corn???

Cooking is one of my hobbies and I am passionate about delicious, wholesome meals made with fresh ingredients. When I eat, I like to enjoy my food and I like to think it is nourishing my body, not poisoning it. I remember buying this cookbook on old style Italian cuisine. I love this cook book so much because it uses such basic, simple ingredients and the food is so delicious. Anyone with minimal skills can cook world class cuisine with a little bit of practice. If you are Italian or if you know an Italian, you know they are passionate about good food. Another observation I made as I flipped through the different sections of this cook book was how far we have strayed in this country from our basic needs to nourish our bodies, to prepackaged convenience foods made by some mad scientists in a lab, manipulated with chemicals, preservatives, food coloring, flash frozen, marketed with a great TV commercial and fancy label and we as consumers are stupid enough to actually pay money for it. I think deep down we all know that this over processed food is not the best for our bodies, but it didn't kill me today like one dose of rat poison so I will eat it again tomorrow. I wonder and you should too, does it............. kill us prematurely over the long haul?????????????????

#8B THE FINANCIAL SIDE

What is obesity costing us in this country? What is it costing us personally? To calculate the financial downside as a country is probably impossible but safe to assume a disastrous amount annually. On a personal level we need to think about a few things. We talked about shopping with a budget, we talked about shopping more conservatively and actually buying what we need instead of what we want. If you saved only 20 dollars per week on a consistent basis, meaning every week of every year, and invested this money ($1000) in your 401k or a mutual fund the long term benefit to your financial situation could be huge!!! I encourage you to contact a financial planner and ask them how much money you will have for retirement if you saved $1000 every year starting right now with compound interest from a 401k plan or a mutual fund. A small family could save even more I bet if you just looked at a few things and were committed to the savings.

I want you to do yourself a favor here. This is an easy way to see how much you are wasting on food every week (this is in addition to the amount that you are over consuming!!!). My simple test is to see how much food you throw out at the end of the week. That's right, how much food goes into the trash at the end of the week, spoiled food, leftovers, stale food, expired food, huge quantities made and only half consumed, huge quantities made, thrown in the freezer, only to be thrown out 6 months later when you clean the freezer because you can't jam any other leftovers in. This was a real eye opener for me when I noticed how much food I was throwing out on a weekly basis. This is when I realized just how much money I was wasting every week or two on groceries by overbuying and not buying/cooking more precisely what was necessary. This savings can be added to if you cut back on the junk food bought during the week at the convenient mart too. Moreover, <u>it is time to cook what you will consume,</u> cooking smaller portions that you will actually eat at one sitting and adjusting your portions to a more sensible size (as I stated earlier, our obesity is a sign of our wealth in this country). I see way too many people cooking for an army when there is only 2!!! If there is a huge amount of mashed potatoes sitting on the table it is too easy to grab another scoop or two. My point is, <u>prepare closer amounts that you will consume comfortably</u> and not leave the table stuffed to the point of discomfort. This may take some time getting use to, <u>getting the portions smaller,</u> but if you pay attention, you can make slight adjustments every meal and get closer every time you cook to minimize the waste and the extra calories. You also need to shop with this minimal attitude. It will change your life.

Another thing I want to mention here is eating should not be a race, especially when eating at home. I think way too many of us consume our food like we are in a race to see who can pork down the most food in the shortest amount of time. If you spent time shopping for the food than preparing it, shouldn't you slow down and enjoy it? I think most people eat so fast they don't even taste their food. Maybe that is why all that garbage food sells, because no one eats slow enough to actually taste how horrible the food they are eating is. If I spend time preparing a balanced meal, I love to sit and enjoy it, I love to taste every bite. My grandparents were European and they enjoyed their meals. Dinner was an event, it was time for conversation, it was time to slow down and reflect, it was time to enjoy the food and the company of others, it was always a feast of hearty home made food, never fast food and never fast paced. My grandparents lived healthy long lives and feasted much. I think there is a good lesson to be learned here...............

#9 HOW TO EASILY MAINTAIN YOUR WEIGHT THROUGHOUT THE HOLIDAYS INSTEAD OF GAINING 5 OR 10 POUNDS

Without a doubt we celebrate the holidays in high style in the U. S. The food, the parties, the gatherings, the shopping, are all signs of our wealth. I know a lot of people gain unwanted pounds over the holiday season and then their New Year's resolution is to lose weight in the new year, exercise more, eat healthier, blahbalahblahhhhhhhhh. For most it has been a new year's resolution for many years (how many years has it been yours?) with very disappointing results. How about a new approach??? Don't gain the weight over the holidays!!! I know for a fact that the pace picks up in most households from mid November through the end of the year. A faster pace should equal weight loss in my book. So where do you go wrong I wonder? I think for most people they go wrong because they don't think. The holidays for most families is a 6 week party/feast. Everywhere you go people have a ton of food, either cooking or buying it. I think the grocery stores see a huge spike in sales around this time. An extra meal here and there (and they usually are large extra meals with lots of calories), extra meals out while shopping, homemade cookies, cakes and treats, and sweets galore. All you have to eat is a few hundred extra calories on average per day throughout the holidays and you can easily gain 5 pounds. I would almost bet most people gain a pound

Thanksgiving week, Christmas week and New Year's week. That's 3 pounds in 3 weeks. My solution and what I practice during the holidays is thinking about the entire week. I make major changes in my eating habits during the holidays. I anticipate the huge, delicious meals by being super conservative throughout the week or skipping a meal here and there so I can pig out (that's right, the master said pig out) on all the delicious foods and not have to worry about gaining one pound throughout the entire holiday season.

Moreover, I can enjoy all the foods, including dessert with no worry of blowing my comfortable weight. <u>It sounds so simple and it is.</u> It kills me when I see people eating like they normally would during the holidays (full breakfasts, etc.) knowing full well they will be starting to cook a feast for one o'clock that day. Eating a huge dinner and still making plans to go out with friends for dinner later that evening. Pigging out at aunt B's knowing they still have to go to gram's for a second courtesy dinner, and you know for sure gram is not going to let you leave until you have to loosen your belt or be rolled out the door into the car (the very worst thing a person can do during their life is eat when they are not hungry, or eat because you are out with friends and they are ordering, or eat because you are bored).

My point here folks is.............. adjust, make changes to your regular schedule, think about your holiday plans and meals, be creative, and make adjustments. Set a goal to maintain your weight through the holidays this year. And fer Christ's sake don't bitch about not being able to eat anything because you are on a strict diet. No one likes to hear a fatty whine about being on a strict diet while they shovel their face with food and sneak sweets all afternoon, it just doesn't look good. <u>You must be more conservative this time of the year during other meals.</u> Go out for dinner fewer times to compensate for the feast. Cut snacks out for 6 weeks so you can enjoy the bounty of the season. If you don't make adjustments and you eat the extra huge meals and enjoy the extra treats on top of your regular food intake like it were a regular week, you will gain weight. And if you think you can take a walk for an hour and offset the feast, wrong again. Smart people learn from their mistakes as well as the mistakes of others. <u>If what you are doing is not working, change what you are doing until you get the desired results.</u> I hope you understand this.

Furthermore, the holidays are usually a very busy time with a faster pace than normal. It should be no problem for most to use this faster pace as an advantage to burn more calories keeping busy and having less time to think about food or snacks between meals, especially if you know you are having a feast that week or that day!!! How stupid do you have to be to eat as if it were a regular day, knowing you were going to sit down to a Christmas day feast with the possibility to consume 2000 calories at one meal??? For most, 2000 calories is enough for the entire day and for some it is even over the limit to maintain proper weight. With that in mind, every single extra calorie you consume that day goes on your body as extra weight. This way of thinking does not only apply to the holidays, it applies to every day of your life. I hope you give this fact serious thought...............

#10 HOW TO AVOID EATING TOO MUCH WHEN YOU GO OUT FOR DINNER AND WHY YOU MUST STOP OR CUT WAY BACK ON GOING TO THE ALL YOU CAN EAT BUFFET

I made this mistake for years while dining out and I bet most people do. Again, I think the way we buy food and go out to eat like there is no tomorrow is a sign of wealth in our country. For most people, we don't have to look at the prices when we are out to eat. We just order what we want and pay the bill at the end (I do wonder if we would order differently if a computer spit out a slip showing the calories, fat, cholesterol, preservatives, food coloring and method of preparation of our order...........). We are hungry and we order with our eyes. Didn't you ever wonder why most restaurants spend all that money on fancy menus with all that fancy camera work? If you just thought about the amount of food you ordered before you ordered you would be ahead of the game here, especially if you are leaving so full you feel sick, it is time to get this handled starting today!!! The expense of dining out these days is something you must think about. You could be throwing away early retirement or the possibility of a financially secure future just by saving a little when you dine out and maybe cutting back on the frequency in which you dine out. Something I did while dining out was instead of me and my lady ordering 2 full meals, we would order one meal and an extra soup or salad and split dinner and maybe order a dessert and split that also. We cut back on our total expense and we still ate well, had a little room for dessert, saved on the overall bill and were not filled to the point of disgust when we left the restaurant. We left satisfied and we saved a few bucks. Our stay was also more enjoyable because we stayed for coffee and dessert on occasion, extending our time and relaxed more and slowed the pace in which we ate. We enjoyed going out to eat more because we changed a few things. We ordered with a plan, we slowed the pace and enjoyed the time together, we had dessert and did not feel guilty about it, and we just enjoyed the overall experience more. We also cut back on our frequency of dining out so it became more of a treat. I really feel if you dine out with too much frequency you lose the feeling that it is a treat that should be enjoyed. Again, this is a sign of our wealth in this country. It is time to look at how many times a week/month you dine out and make some adjustments. [Just a few thoughts how couples can save calories and money, and still enjoy going out for dinner without eating like a pig and wasting money.]

[tangent] Recently while dining out with a buddy I made a huge discovery. We were at a nice restaurant and we ordered seafood. My dinner came with a small fork stuck in my lemon. I think they are called cocktail forks or seafood forks. This fork was about 75% smaller than a regular dinner fork and I decided to eat my meal with it instead of the usual American size dinner fork (I ordered a lobster tail with vegetables and mashed potatoes just to give you an idea what was on my plate). We were chatting and eating and having a good time and joking about the tiny fork I was using. Now, here is what I discovered. Half way through our meal my friend had already consumed his mashed potatoes, and mine were only about a third gone. I remember looking over and saying to him, "Dude, your potatoes are all gone!", and I noticed the huge amount of potatoes he had on his fork as he ate the last bite, probably 4 or 5 times the quantity I was getting on my tiny fork!!! Furthermore, I noticed something else that may be the biggest lesson in this course and I must tell you it even opened up my eyes again to new areas that we all can improve upon in our daily eating habits. What I noticed was

my friend was consuming a huge fork full of potatoes each time he loaded his fork and moved it to his mouth. My tiny fork could only hold 25% of what I would usually load on my regular size dinner fork, but here is another amazing discovery.............. <u>I was enjoying the smaller portion of the potatoes much more,</u> I was more able to taste the smaller portion in my mouth as I chewed them, rather than having a huge fork full in my mouth and unable to fully taste the large portion. I feel we chew a little and because we are in such a hurry we then swallow the glut of quantity in our mouth so we can <u>taste</u> another bite as quickly as possible. These were not the best mashed potatoes I have ever had in my life, but I did enjoy them more than I have ever enjoyed mashed potatoes in my life and I must say it was the tiny portion in my mouth that made all the difference. I hope you are getting this!!! Moreover, as I ate my vegetables I noticed the smaller portions also tasted better and as I sliced my lobster tail and could only get so much on my tiny fork, I was able to fully enjoy and taste it, too. Lobster tail is one of my favorite foods to eat and believe me if I could get a whole tail on a fork I would eat it in one bite. But my point is I wouldn't have been able to fully enjoy and taste every morsel of my lobster tail or any other part of my meal as much, until I discovered just how much more I could taste and fully enjoy the smaller portions I was putting on my tiny fork. You must try this test yourself. Try putting smaller portions (75% less than normal) on your fork and see how much better you can taste and enjoy your food. I did not feel deprived as I ate either. I was totally happy with the fact the tiny portions tasted so good, plus the time to eat my meal was longer as I ate slower and took many more fork fulls than normal. After a good 20 or 30 minutes at the restaurant, I was pleasantly full and did not feel like a stuffed pig. I had little to no desire for dessert as my stomach had plenty of time to signal my brain that we were full and all was well and happy down here.

See, this is not about willpower here folks (very few people in this world will ever win the battle with will power alone). This is about making a little discovery that can change your eating habits and way of life forever for the better and not be starving yourself and not feel deprived at the dinner table. At this point I wonder if I should be designing an entire new set of cutlery and dinner plates and even glasses for everyday home use. Think about it, our forks, spoons, knives, dishes and glasses are huge. As I said, the larger the portion we have the more we are going to eat. I don't care if it is a huge cereal box, a 2 liter bottle of soda and a 16 ounce glass or a huge dinner plate that will hold enough food for 2 persons. The more quantity we have, the more we will eat!!! I encourage everyone to think about this section a lot and try some tests yourself and see how you feel and what you discover.

#10A THE ALL YOU CAN EAT BUFFET

Now maybe I don't know nothin about nothin, but if you have a weight problem, why on earth would you be going to the all you can eat buffet? I know people that count every calorie at every meal all week long then go to the all you can eat buffet once a week or once a month as a social event or because it is a good deal and they can't figure out why they can't get their weight under control. The all you can eat buffet is not a good deal!!! It is a bad deal!!! Let's think about it. You pay one price and you can eat like a pig, you can eat as much as you like for as long as you like or until you bust out of your pants. These places are not a good deal. You can easily pork on 2000 calories (because you can't control yourself) you do not need.

Even if you only go once a month for a treat (yeah right) you can gain an easy 5 pounds over the year and that is if every other day throughout the year your diet and exercise program is perfect. The last time I went was about 6 years ago and I found a few things of interest. [I don't see myself going back to any buffet in the near future or maybe this lifetime.] #1 The food was terrible. There was quantity and selection but no quality in my book. #2 I saw enough obese people at this place to make me never want to go back again. #3 Personally, I found the whole experience sad and disgusting. The only reason these places survive is because of human nature, you pay one price and you can eat as much as you want. You know the food is not that good, you know you eat way to much, you know it probably isn't that great for you, but you keep going back because it is a good deal. Not!!! Maybe it is time you got with the program here. Think about something. If you went shopping at the mall and it cost $20.00 and they gave you a small plastic bag and they said you can have whatever you can stuff in the bag, would you get what you needed or would you leave the mall with that bag bulging at the seams? It is the same with the buffet, you paid one price and you eat until you are bulging at the seams. It is simply human nature to get or eat as much as you can if you pay one price. You feel like s..., but boy did we get our money's worth. That way of thinking will have you obese.

#11 HOW TO HANDLE THE UNEXPECTED LUNCH OR DINNER DATE WHEN YOU'RE NOT HUNGRY

Did you ever just think of saying no? I am in business and I have plenty of colleagues and friends with flexible schedules that often call or invite me out for dinner or lunch. When I was figuring things out I was very concerned if the occasional, unplanned dinner date would throw my plan off course. What I discovered is if it were only occasionally I was OK, but if it got too frequent it was no good. I needed to think about this more and I came up with a plan, especially if I was not hungry or not planning on eating anything else that day. My first approach was flat out telling someone that I had just ate and I was not interested in dinner that eve or lunch that day. If it was a business meeting, I would hold it at my office instead of meeting at a restaurant.

As I said people respect people with some self control. I get a lot of respect because I display discipline. Sometimes there is the unavoidable lunch date that just doesn't fit your day and some people do a lot of business over lunch or in restaurants. If it is a business lunch that you have to go to, the easiest thing I do is focus on business and not the food. Order light with this in mind and do not drink alcohol. You must be professional and being in control is mandatory here. Focus on the conversation, focus on business and eat very slow and order something easy to eat or pick at.

I remember practicing these techniques and barely touching my food throughout the entire meal and not even missing it as the waitress takes it away. If you focus on the conversation/business you will be able to pick at your food with very little worry about eating too much. When out with friends it is no different, you must show some discipline. If you know that you will be eating later or you have already eaten what is necessary for the day you must think about this and realize any extra calories you eat at this sitting are going to add to your weight. This is an area for some self evaluation. See how many times a week or month these situations arise and see how you normally handle them. You can also think about the unwanted calories you are porking on during these times. If it is a rare occasion I wouldn't worry too much, but if you think it is adding to your troubles you must take action and make adjustments.

#12 UNDERSTANDING CALORIES AND FOOD

In my opinion there is a huge difference between calories and food. In section 13 we talk about a 2000 calorie per day diet and just how few calories that is per day. Now, if you do major hard physical labor during the day at your job, your daily allowance will be higher and I highly recommend you figure out real closely how many calories you are burning on a consistent basis per week as mentioned in section 13. <u>It is extremely important you have a feel for how many calories per day you burn.</u> After you have this figured out you can divide your calories needed per day by how many meals you eat per day and have a really good idea where you are running into problems and why you are overweight. Obviously, if you want to start losing weight you will have to eat fewer calories per day on a consistent basis to start this process (refer to section 2A).

Here is where I think many get into trouble. First off, people don't realize how few calories are required throughout the day to keep your body healthy, slim, and satisfied. Let's use a general example and say after you figure out your daily calories needed it is 2000 for easy figuring, and you eat 3 meals per day. That = about 650 calories per meal that you can consume and not gain anymore weight. Again, this is not many calories!!! Now, each person must think about what they normally eat at meal time. If you don't have a clue the calories in the foods you are eating, I highly recommend you go to the book store and get a calorie pocket manual that lists most foods you consume so you can get an idea just how many calories you are consuming per meal. This is very important.

Once you start taking notice of the calories in different foods I think you will be shocked like I was just how much difference there is between food and calories in the things we shove in our mouths. I consider food the good stuff (meat, fruit and vegetables) and I consider calories the bad stuff (junk food, fast food, soda, and snacks). The point I want you to get here is that if you only have 650 calories to blow per meal you don't want to be getting those calories in the form of a soda and a muffin at the convenient mart, or a microwave sandwich and a power drink, and you certainly don't want to be blowing half of your calories at a fast food joint getting a greasy double cheeseburger, fries and a soda (a fast food lunch can easily be 1000 calories). You just have blown half of your calories for the day with very little nutrition for your body. The worst part is you now only have 1000 calories left for the entire day to try to get something healthy into your body. That leaves you with 2 meals of only 500 calories each. I think if you came home for dinner and you had 500 calories of good food on your plate you would actually freak out when you saw just how small the portions were. If you went out to dinner and were served these small portions on a 6 inch plate I am certain you would walk out and never return.

I will attempt to paint you a picture of 500 calories of food for dinner. 4 to 5 ounces of meat which is about 9 bites depending if it was chicken or steak, about 8 tablespoons of peas or other greens in similar portions, and about 6 tablespoons of mashed potatoes. Give or take a little. <u>My point here is 500 calories is hardly anything!!!</u> Now you can throw all your large dinner plates in the garbage because this meal will fit on a 6 inch plate. And yes, you will be having ice water with dinner tonight honey. No soda, not a six pack of beer, no milk, no coffee, no juice, no tea, no bread, no butter, no sauces or gravies, no dessert later, no chocolate <u>and certainly no snacks for TV time!!!</u> I hope you get the picture here!!! Now let's think about a dinner out. Let's go for a 12 ounce prime rib, a baker with butter and sour cream, a vegetable, loads of free bread and soup or salad for starters and ice water as a drink. I am using rounded average figures here just to give you an idea of a common dinner out. I am going to throw a round number out there of 1500 to 2000 calories for a dinner like this. You can easily eat your entire daily requirements for calories in one dinner or lunch out in a restaurant. Keep in mind we had ice water and no dessert or cocktails.

I really think restaurants should post calories and fat on their menu items. I think most people would be shocked at just how many calories they consume when eating out. If you threw on a few drinks, dessert, and coffee on the above dinner which most people do, you can easily see how you can get into the 2000 to 2500 range very easily. Shocking?

The point that I want you to think about in this section is to start to separate the healthy and nutritious foods that your body is dying for, from the huge calorie/fat junk food that does nothing for your body except pack on the pounds and leaves your body starving for nutrition and balance. I think if most people took what they consumed over the period of a month and did a food pyramid like we did in the 3rd grade. Most would be shocked how little nutrition they ate and how much poison they poured into their bodies. I think the modern day food pyramid would be saturated fat, cholesterol, sugar, salt, preservatives, artificial flavors, artificial sweeteners, artificial color, and in the very bottom with the smallest percentage would be healthy nutritious foods. Furthermore, I feel most people have no balance in their diets at all.

#13 WHY MOST PEOPLE CAN'T EAT 3 BIG MEALS PER DAY AND WHY YOU CAN'T SNACK BETWEEN MEALS, WHILE DRIVING, WHEN WATCHING TV, OR LATE AT NIGHT JUST BEFORE NIGHTNIGHT

In my opinion, most people cannot eat 3 big meals a day like people did 50 years ago. Most people do not burn enough calories during the day doing their modern day cushy jobs to justify 3 meals a day plus the undisciplined snacks, soda, and pure junk food. It seems like we have forgot about all the good stuff from 50 years ago except the 3 meals per day for everyone. I hate to break the bad news to you, but most people don't deserve 3 big meals a day and obviously our bodies are telling us the same thing by being obese. Being obese for most people is their body's way of telling them you are shoving too much food down us that we have no need for and the only thing we can do with it is store it as fat on your gut and your butt. 50 years ago people worked hard at their jobs and around the home and could easily justify 3 hearty meals per day (they were burning a lot more calories!!!) and if you watch old movies or look at old pictures from that era people were very slim. Also, people cooked more meals and they did not have tons of snacks and practically no junk food lying around in every corner and cupboard to pig out on. People ate 3 meals a day because they were burning that many calories during their normal day and it shows they were in balance with their body's demands and needs by being fairly slim, and in my opinion, more healthy. Back then if you wanted something to eat you had to make it and it required more effort than going to the freezer and microwaving some nasty snack or grabbing a bag of cookies or chips. How much late night snacking would you do if it required great effort and time to prepare? Seeing how lazy we are I would say little or none. You know the term sweet treat? Did you ever take 2 seconds to think about its meaning? To me, a sweet is cake, donuts, ice cream, cookies, or pastry (even soda). It is a treat because you don't have it all the time and usually on special occasions only. I remember when I was growing up, and this is only about 25 years ago, but we did not have candy, cake, donuts or cookies filling the countertop or cupboards at home. That is why we called them sweet treats. Furthermore, we did not have a freezer full of junk foods that you could microwave.

I really feel <u>everyone</u> must figure out on average how many calories <u>they</u> burn on a daily basis during the week and per weekend and get a solid daily/weekly average. In a nutshell, average males should eat around 2000 calories per day and average women should eat about 1500 calories per day. Most packaging says daily values based on a 2000 calorie diet. In my opinion you cannot be this general with something so important. Go online and figure out exactly what your body type needs on a daily basis to maintain your weight. If you are off by only 100 calories per day (which is nothing) you will gain 10 unwanted pounds in only one year. Unchecked for 5 years and you are a whopping 50 pounds overweight and obese. It is impossible for me to go into great detail about every person's daily needs, but what you can do is go online and enter your age, weight, height and gender on a calorie calculator WEBSITE and it will show you calculations of calories burned for different activities during the day so you can calculate a very accurate number of calories required by your body to maintain a healthy weight and lifestyle. <u>This simple test will show you why you are overweight.</u> It will show you how few calories we burn in our cushy lifestyle on a daily basis. I think it will open your eyes and be one of those moments when the lights go on and you say I have been sold a bill of goods that just does not work anymore and are not accurate anymore <u>and I must adjust my way of thinking today and from this day forward.</u> Another thing we must think about. Even if we are burning 2000 calories per day that it is really not that many calories and it leaves little room for error and <u>no room for snacks.</u> Take 2000 calories and divide by 3 meals. That = only 666 calories per meal. I hope you can start to see where we are getting into trouble here. 666 calories is not much of a meal and that is 0 calories for snacks, sweets, soda, and junk food between meals. I heard someone say you should eat 5 meals per day to keep your metabolism high, I would like to know what you could eat at 400 calories per meal and consider it a meal. At 400 calories per meal it is not worth getting the dish dirty.

Another point here is, keep your diet secrets to yourself. Once you understand this course and you start using the secrets that work for you and you start shaping up and feeling better and your clothes fit better, keep what works to yourself and <u>be careful of well meaning obese friends offering their advice about the last 100 quick fix diets they have tried</u> and why they all failed. Be polite, nod your head and yaddaaayyaadddaaa and just remember that there is no quick fix and your eyes have been opened to the simple facts. <u>And remember just how delicate a balance it is between a healthy, comfortable weight and obesity.</u>

#14 POISON VS. FOOD

Throughout the course I talk about poison and food and I just want to make a few points here. In my opinion food is what is required by your body to function properly and maintain a healthy weight. Poison (not like rat poison, one dose and you are out) is basically anything not needed to maintain proper weight and health. But I do consider food that has been over processed/preserved and chemically manipulated by a mad scientist to be poison and over long periods of time does harm our bodies. I will also tell you I am not a fan of junk foods or soda, and I don't care if it is diet soda either. I feel they bring nothing to the party except obesity and a plethora of other health problems.

I think every person should get a piece of paper and do this little exercise. The exercise is to draw a line down the center of a piece of paper. At the top of the left column write food (<u>nutritious food</u> would even be better to write here), and at the top of the right column write poison. Now I want you to start writing down what you eat on a daily/weekly/monthly basis in the proper column. This exercise can be done over the course of a month if you really want to get the most accurate account of exactly what you are putting in your body. You must be honest with yourself here and use your best judgment on placing everything you eat in the proper column. I think this will open your eyes and make you see that the poison column outweighs the food column way too much. I recommend you keep this list and I also recommend you start adjusting this list to get more on the food side and less on the poison side. I highly recommend you draw a line through some of the poison foods and either eliminate them completely from your diet or severely limit their consumption. At minimum, I feel this quick exercise will open your eyes and show you that you have plenty of room for improvement. You may want to redo the list 6 months from now and review your improvements. These changes must be made for the rest of your life.

Personally, what I found was that the fresh food tastes so much better than the junk food it is easy to change, if you just think about it.............. Get a visual of a junk food factory, a huge vat of this sludge being mixed with a huge bag of secret mystery powder combined with a huge tank of liquid food coloring/corn syrup and recycled plant water baked in a 600 degree oven to kill everything, extruded into bite size flavor enhanced pieces, packaged in a fancy bag and boom you have the perfect junk food. Let's not forget the mad plant owner screaming, "More-more-more, more production, more money, more fat people!!!", laughing all the way to the bank with no concern for you or your health. After all, the ___ approved all these wonder ingredients and they are perfectly safe for high consumption in lab rats, oops, I mean people. [Did you ever wonder just how long those lab rats live? I have wondered if they live long enough to see the long term effects or do they drop dead prematurely of obesity or cancer.............. Just something to think about.] Then 20 years later you read in the paper, darn we got this one wrong and we need to pull this or that off the shelves because those rats all did die. All the consumer gets is the 'oh well' shrug from the manufacturer and the ___ and the better luck next time attitude. Maybe it is time we all thought about this more, maybe it is time to leave the rat food for the rats, maybe this thought alone will help you change your eating habits and stop you from grabbing the rat food, junk food, and all the other unnecessary poison calories..............

Another thought I had and wanted to share. Nicotine, sugar and salt. [The definition of nicotine from a college dictionary. A colorless, oily, water soluble, highly toxic alkaloid found in tobacco and valued as an insecticide. It does not mention anything about being addictive.? Maybe a few key words used in the definition will help some people kick the bad habit? Highly toxic and valued as an

54

insecticide.? HELLO!!!] I think it is pretty safe to say that nicotine has an addictive quality and as bad as smoking is people cannot kick the bad habit because their bodies crave the nicotine. My thought is, I wonder if sugar and salt also have an addictive quality, or do they create a craving in our bodies that drive us to consume the salty snacks, sweets, soda and junk food even though we know it is not good for our bodies. This is a question we must all ask ourselves. Without a doubt the tobacco companies have made a fortune with their product and our wonderful government has raked in huge tax dollars, too. I wonder if the fast food and junk food industry have been raking in the coin with a similar approach? What do you think?

[story time] Have you ever heard the old saying, you can lead a horse to water but you can't make him drink? Well I don't agree with that saying. Because if you give a horse a nice salty bag of oats you can make him drink almost every time............... Anyway, what to do? My advice is to start to wean yourself off of these products slowly, <u>start lowering the amount that you consume,</u> and gradually I feel most can kick the habit. And I don't care if it is smoking or eating to much junk food/poison, salt, sugar or nicotine.

A freebie for smokers (and all can use this analogy to their benefit). I feel if a smoker took this 12 month approach, most could quit smoking by breaking the dependency, by weaning their bodies from craving nicotine. When people try to quit smoking cold turkey, I feel most fail because the bodies craving for nicotine is so high (and not necessarily the cigarette itself or the smoking of that nasty thing) it will overrule the willpower of a person most of the time. Cravings are very, very powerful. My advice for smokers would be to take their cigarettes and measure the smokeable portion and divide that number by 12 months and record these figures. For easy figuring lets say the smokeable area is 3 inches long. That means you will be cutting each cigarette by 1/4 of an inch in length each month for one year. Every month for one year I recommend that you cut each cigarette that you would smoke per month shorter in length according to your calculations (you must smoke the same number of packs that you would normally be smoking per month!!!). Each month your cigarettes will keep getting shorter and shorter and be giving your body <u>slightly</u> less nicotine per month. By the end of the 12 months there will be no cigarette length to smoke. At this point I hope your body is not craving the nicotine. I hope when you start to think about the wasted money, the wasted years of your life, the foul smelling breath, the foul smell in your clothes and vehicle and your home, it will be enough leverage on your side to kick the habit forever and <u>change your identity into being a non-smoker.</u> As I said, you can use this same weaning off approach in other areas of your life, whether it be a bad habit like smoking or a bad habit of eating too much food or junk food.

Enough. Let's move on to greener pastures. Food to me is fresh food that you buy in the produce aisle or at the meat counter at the grocery store, fresh baked breads, unprocessed fruits and vegetables, milk and eggs, fresh meats and seafood, and natural fruit juices and teas. As you can see this is not a huge selection, and as you observe the next time you go shopping it is only about 20% of the shelf space. But I will guarantee you the combinations with these few selections can have you eating great tasting healthy and nutritious foods with very little repetition throughout the year. I challenge you to buy an old world cookbook and see how simple the recipes are and how basic the ingredients and how great the food tastes. I have cooked much for many years and it is rare that a recipe calls for more than basic ingredients. I never once went to a lab and bought wonder powder to cook with or added any of those other lab created ingredients found in most junk food that you can't pronounce.

#15 LOSING THE SCALE AND THE DISAPPOINTMENT

In section 28 I talk about when I was busting out of my size 32 waist jeans and when I started figuring this whole weight gain/loss problem out I did not have a scale in my house. To this day I still do not have a scale in my house and I really don't care how much I weigh as long as my 32-32 jeans fit well and I am happy with the way I feel and look. [I am sure my weight fluctuates a few pounds throughout the year but I do not stress over it. To me it is all about wearing the same size jeans for the rest of my life and fitting in them comfortably and feeling good about myself, knowing I have beat the diet roller coaster ride.] It seems to me that most everyone has a scale in their bathroom and they weigh in every morning but it does not seem to be having any positive effect on their weight control. <u>Furthermore, the massive number of people that do weigh in everyday and see their weight on the rise and they don't take action to change course is totally amazing to me!!!</u> I am talking about intelligent people here!!! I ask you, how can you consider yourself an intelligent person when month after month you see another pound adding on to your weight and you don't change something in your lifestyle to stop this from happening? Look, if you want to be fat and happy that is fine with me, but if you are concerned about your weight and your health, how can you continue the same patterns and still consider yourself and intelligent life form? Do you know enough to come in out of the rain?

Another interesting thing I want to discuss here is that weighing yourself in the AM and knowing the needle just keeps rising higher on the scale, it just isn't powerful enough to control our food intake throughout the day. People are weak in this country. We have little or no self control and I think the mindset is, well, I will eat more sensibly tomorrow or the next day or next week I will get serious, but next week never comes and the weight packs on. Nobody balloons out in a week, but gone unchecked over a year or even 5 years a person can really pork on the pounds. Weighing in in the AM is an interesting process too, like the only hope people have is to lose weight while they sleep because they didn't feed their fat face while they slept and when they wake and weigh in maybe a miracle happened while they slept (I am sure that will be the next magic pill offer, slim down while you sleep).

I can't drive this point home enough so here I go again. <u>There is no quick fix, maintaining a comfortable/healthy weight is a way of live, every minute of everyday for the rest of your life you have to think before you eat.</u> Perhaps you should try putting the scale in the closet and just start applying things you learned in this course and start adjusting your weight slowly but surely and stop being disappointed in the short term and let the long term handle itself. I feel strongly that people are expecting overnight results and they want to check their progress everyday. I also feel the average home scale is not even accurate enough to sense the small loss or gain on a daily basis, therefore it only adds to the roller coaster ride. I know some people get so frustrated when they weigh in in the AM, so they just pig out at breakfast and say to hell with it out of frustration.

Again, it goes back to the way we have been brain washed by the bombardment of ads everywhere we turn for the fast, quick and easy weight loss magic pill, potion or equipment. One of the most important things I can tell you is <u>you must stop thinking there is a magic quick fix.</u> When you understand this it will change your way of thinking and may be the break through that will change your way of life forever. The day you break the cycle, break away from your past bad habits, you will be on your way to solving your weight problems forever. Once you gain control and feel the power of being in control, it will change your life. Maybe you need to jam this thought in your brain. From today forward for the rest of my life I will not be a sucker anymore, I will never be ripped off ever again with a quick fix quack remedy, from today forward I will be a more disciplined person!!! I feel everyone can benefit from being a more disciplined person in many areas of their lives. Start today and see major results in all areas of your life by being more disciplined.

#16 GETTING TO THE ROOT OF THE PROBLEM

As discussed in section #2, I feel there are only 2 simple ways to adjust your weight, and they are eating less or burning more calories. I feel it is time we got to the root of the problem here. We have talked about exercise and being more active and our lazy/comfy lifestyles and all the modern conveniences and gadgets we have invented in this country to make our lives easy. Now, don't get me wrong here. Exercise and being active is a very important part of being healthy, but I think a lot of people exercise (for all the wrong reasons) to burn off the extra food they eat so they don't become obese. In my opinion this is for the wrong reason and not getting to the root of the problem. I have seen way too many people join gyms, clubs, organizations, buy expensive exercise equipment and it is great for a while, but then slowly they get tired of working out or they get bored at the gym. You get the picture. I am sure many of you have been there, done that, too.............. <u>My point here is very important. If you're not going to stick with the gym or the exercise equipment for the rest of your life, it is not going to solve your long term weight issues.</u>

This course is not a quick fix. It is designed to make you think differently from today forward and make life long changes so you can get to a healthy weight and maintain it for the rest of your life. <u>The essence of getting to the root of the problem is understanding that</u>

you must control the amount of food you eat everyday for the rest of your life to maintain your comfortable weight. If you are eating too much on a regular basis and off setting it by a one year membership at the gym that you will not renew, what happens then? You spin out of control. You pork on the extra pounds and you are screwed. Don't get me wrong here folks. If you are going to go to the gym or use the treadmill for the rest of your life and it works for you, you are golden, but I know the majority will not stick with the exercise for a lifetime.

[a little story] I remember going fishing with a friend some years ago and we had to get up at like 4 AM to get ready because it was a long drive to the lake. Now for most people, including myself, it would take a pack of wild horses to get them out of bed at 4 AM, but if you are passionate about something and really enjoy doing it, it is no problem. Did you ever know someone who was passionate about a hobby and just loved doing it and just couldn't wait to get to it? The point. If you have to force yourself to work out or go to the gym it is only a matter of time before you stop. On the other hand, if you are passionate about working out you have a chance of sticking with it. As I discussed in section 6, I discovered I love being outside, hiking in the woods, cutting wood and cleaning my property, planting trees, walking the trails for hours being in nature. Not only did I benefit from the exercise, but the peace I got from being outside in nature and destressing after a week of working in the city is priceless for me!!! This is what I discovered I love doing and I have a passion for it and I see myself doing this for the rest of my life because I love it so much and I know the huge benefits to my body and overall well being. Bottom line, discover what activity or hobby you can get passionate about and stick with for a long time or even the rest of your life.

#17 ABOUT 300 MILLION PEOPLE IN THE U. S. AND ABOUT 6 BILLION ON PLANET EARTH

Focusing on the U. S. population, I was thinking about the round number of 300 million people. What came to mind was 300 million people of what size and consuming how much? I'm just throwing some numbers out here, but if we are as a whole consuming 15% more due to our size as in being obese and consuming more than the necessary calories of 1500 to 2000 per day on average, for a slim person we are looking at a huge difference in consumption. If I use a conservative figure of 15% excess consumption, that is roughly equal to having another 50 million people in the U. S. alone. This equals a huge drain on our resources and a huge amount of extra garbage in our landfills and pollution in our air and water. The obesity problem is more far reaching than most think. It is much more severe than not fitting in your clothes or ruining your health. If we start putting dollar signs on the problem in the U. S. alone it would be a devastating figure. If we start to think about the extra production in our factories, which equals huge amounts of energy consumed and the pollution from the factories and the delivery trucks alone, you can see the negative effects of excessive consumption, the drain of overworking our farmland to feed an obese nation. A wise man once said, "A nation that over works its soil and pollutes its waters has no future." Just something to think about.............. Lately we have all been doing our part recycling our trash in an effort to not pollute our soil and water with more landfills. Without a doubt it is a good idea, but doing your part may boil down to something very simple with a far more reaching benefit and that is, not consuming so damn much like there is no tomorrow. This is not only with food either. We seem to be shoppers of excess in all areas of our lives, buying things on sale that we really don't need (ladies), buying imported junk from you know where that fails after the second use or does not work like the TV ad showed, and we store it in the garage or simply throw it out with the 'oh well' attitude. If we calculated the money we wasted as a nation on excess food and junk products we don't need, in one year we could probably pay off the national debt!!!

Another bone I want to pick here is our approach in how we fix things in this nation. It never seems anyone wants to get to the root of the problem. It's like instead of getting to the root of the problem we like to put bandaids on things or we take the after the fact approach. If we got to the root of the obesity problem as in stop eating so much there would be no industry building all these workout gadgets (less pollution, less consumption of resources) sold by gorgeous movie stars that most blow their money on, use for a few months and then slide them into the closet or basement never to be used again, or blown out at a garage sale for 10 cents on the dollar. That equals 90% of your hard earned money wasted. We seem to like to take the after the fact approach in this country because it is way more profitable for somebody I guess. Unfortunately, I feel the consumer is the biggest loser here and big companies the big winner. After the fact to me is, eat like a pig then buy this gadget to burn the calories off. After the fact to me is, eat more than your body needs and pop this magic pill that may or may not work. The fact is, you are eating more than your body needs. Not getting to the root of the problem to me is, putting a bucket in your living room to catch the rainwater from a leaky roof, instead of repairing the roof. Our over consumption in this country (in all areas of our lives!!!) is having a huge and far reaching negative effect that I don't think most people want to be made aware of (I'm not going to get into global warming or soaring healthcare here).

The main reason for writing this section was to make people aware of the fact that we are over consuming in all areas of our lives and I feel it is having a very negative effect not only on our quality of life but on our country as a whole and even on our planet. 300 million bodies compared to consuming like 350 million is a huge difference and a huge extra burden on the planet, I feel. Recycling is a feel good thing and I agree it's a start but let's slow down on the over consumption like there is no tomorrow, because if we don't slow down, there may not be another tomorrow 94 years from now...............

#18 EATING THE FOODS YOU LOVE

Personally, I never deprive myself of the foods that I love. The only thing that comes to mind that I really don't enjoy is cucumbers. Anything else is fair game in my book. I can't stand low fat or low calorie foods and I hate diet soda. In my opinion, diet soda should never have been invented!!! I believe it was created because people love the taste of soda so much, but when they started seeing how much they consumed on a weekly basis they knew they were gaining weight just because of the extra calories in the soda alone. Now comes along some smart businessman realizing if he could create some type of sweetener that had only a mildly foul taste and shoved it in soda, people would buy it like there was no tomorrow and he would be very rich. Wow wee!!! All the taste (to me it has a foul taste that I can't stand) and no calories, and sure enough the diet soda business is a huge success and is super profitable. The way I see people at the grocery store loading their carts with soda like they were preparing for Armageddon, it has to be huge business.

My point here is a few regular tasty sodas a week should not be a problem, we can enjoy regular soda just like everything else but it must be in moderation. To me, soda is a treat, not a life sustaining necessity. Whatever happened to regular old ice water to quench your thirst and hydrate your cells? This is what your body needs, not sugar water with caramel coloring. Whatever happened to regular old moo cow milk that actually came from a cow and not a soybean? Hello.............. Whatever happened to real 100% fruit juices? I love iced teas with no sugar added and brewed by the sun as in solar tea. Good taste and 0 calories.

This whole section is about moderation. The U. S. seems to be the land of excess and we need to start thinking and eating differently. As far as the low cal or no cal food goes, I would rather eat a little less of the real thing that actually has taste than a large amount of the tasteless low cal that has been created in a lab by scientists. I just don't feel your body knows what to do with those chemicals or sugar substitutes that are put in these foods, and I don't want to think of the potential long term negative side effects of consuming these foods in quantity. What I do know, is these large companies that make the diet sodas and all the other low cal food are making a huge profit on the consumer and I don't see it having much effect on the battle of the bulge. Maybe it is time you ask yourself the same question I did a long time ago. Is this low cal food where it's at or is it killing me slowly but surely? It all goes back to human nature and people not being able to control the quantity of food they eat. It is further multiplied with our cushy jobs and lifestyles and it goes back to the U. S. being a wealthy nation that doesn't have to think about every penny they spend on food. If we were dirt poor like other nations and we had to account for every last penny we spent on food I think we would not be an obese nation and we would have no need for diet soda or low fat food with no taste. The mentality is I can eat twice as much low cal food for the same calories and I can pour down as many of these diet sodas as I like because they don't have one calorie. I hate to break the bad news to you but it is a totally wrong mindset that must be changed. I guess I have beat up enough on the diet soda and low cal foods and I hope you take a good look in your refrigerator and make some adjustments. I hope you think about natural foods vs. synthetic-science-lab-food creations.

As you know by now I love to cook and I love to eat. I feel it is almost impossible to eliminate a food you love from your diet completely and I feel almost 90% of the diets that say you can eat all the salad you like or you can eat as much cabbage soup as you can pour down or the all you can eat protein diets don't work long term. I have seen people on these diets and they drive themselves crazy depriving themselves of the foods they love. I have seen the above diets work short term but with little success over the long term. The base of these all you can eat diets is just that, all you can eat without any self control on quantity. Anyone that tries these diets has not got a grip on the fact that you can't eat unlimited quantities of anything. I don't care if they are organic carrots. You have not got to the root of the problem and the root of the problem is you do have to limit the calories you eat everyday for the rest of your life. [If you learn only one thing from reading this material, I hope it is the fact of just how delicate a balance it is between being healthy and fit and being obese and having health issues. You must get some kind of control in your life starting today!!!] I have never seen one person I know that tried the all you can eat salad or protein diet stick with it long term.

On the surface, nothing seems better than eat as much steak, eggs, and cheese as you can handle. I have seen it work short term, people lose weight and they look great and then you see them a year later and they look like ..... They gained every pound back and you ask them, like gee, what happened? The usual response I got from people that tried the all you can eat protein diet was, "I just got sick and tired of it.............. I craved bread, I craved fruit, I craved sweets, I craved pastries, the cravings drove me nuts, I could not stick with it for the rest of my life, so I bagged the whole concept." I have personally seen people on the protein diet that would have climbed a barbed wire fence for a piece of bread or a piece of fruit. I deprive myself of nothing!!! I love a full breakfast with bacon, eggs, homefries or hash, toast with real butter and jelly, fresh milk and juice, but it is only on occasion that I have it and it's a treat that I thoroughly enjoy. Moreover, when I do make the full blown breakfast, I make huge adjustments to the amount of food I consume during lunch and dinner. Sometimes I will even skip lunch because breakfast was so hearty and I don't even miss it. And I don't make the full blown breakfast with a full blown dinner ever in the same day. That would be way too many calories. On the weekends I love cooking full blown world class cuisine for lunch or dinner with roasted meats, fish, grilled steaks or chops, fresh vegetables, potatoes made with butter and breads and even jelly donuts, cheesecake or full fat ice cream for my sweet treat. I take the leftovers to lunch during the week and I get great tasting, nutritious food and it keeps me away from the fast food joints and the microwave convenient mart foods and junk foods. And yes, I still fit comfortably in my 32-32 jeans.

I bet some of you are reading the above foods that I love and are saying, "Boy, I wish I could enjoy those foods." The fact is, most people can enjoy rich foods like I do, too, but it must be in moderation and it must be with a plan. I go shopping with a plan and you must too. I don't buy the donuts, ice cream, or cake every week. As I mentioned these are my sweet treats that maybe I eat once every 3 or 4 months and in small portions. When I buy ice cream it is in the premium selection and in very small quantities, not the 2 gallon pail size that sits in the freezer so it can be eaten every night while watching the late show. I may buy ice cream only once or twice a year, but I can enjoy it without guilt and without killing my heart. If you buy ice cream or any food in the 2 gallon pail size, those days are over. Moreover, I feel the bulk packaging and super size packaging was one of the worst concepts ever developed from an obese nation point of view. I just feel the more we have the more we eat and that is where we are getting in trouble. Excessive buying and excessive consumption.

The Europeans have been enjoying rich foods and it seems like they have very little weight problems and a lot less health problems. Their rate of heart disease is staggeringly lower than the U. S., as well as other diseases. If you are thin and lean your body functions like a well oiled machine and everything hums along in harmony, but when you start to get heavy or obese, your organs have to work much harder to perform their jobs. Think of your body like an overloaded truck climbing a steep hill on a hot summer day, the engine being your heart. If you keep pushing with the heavy load the engine will overheat, like a mild heart attack. If you keep pushing without lightening up the load you run the risk of complete failure of your engine or a heart that explodes from being overworked and under appreciated.

#19 SERVING SIZES, THEN AND NOW

In continuing in sorts with section 18, we must look at serving sizes 50 or even 20 years ago vs. the modern day super size portions. The portions that are put in front of us today are simply out of control!!! I remember watching this show on bagels and it showed over the years how a bagel went from its original size of about 3 inches in diameter to our modern day super size of nearly double, or 5 to 6 inches in diameter. It's not just bagels either. Basically everything that is marketed to us has grown in size over the last 20 years. I call it one-up marketing by big companies. Like if my burger joint was offering a normal 8 ounce soda with a meal and my competitor started offering a 12 ounce drink for the same price to grab all my customers, it is a form of marketing. When word got around that joint A was offering a larger soda for the same price, it would cause an increase in business. Most customers would go for the larger quantity of soda because it seemed like they were getting a better deal. Larger quantity for the same price = good deal in most peoples heads. Now, after awhile when burger joint A's sales started slipping he would offer a 16 ounce drink and a few more fries to try to lure his customers back, and so we start a viscous cycle of one-up marketing (I call it). This is my theory on how we went from a normal 8 ounce serving size drink to a 16 ounce or I have seen as high as a 32 ounce jumbo size. Take a look at the coolers in the stores with the drinks in them. How many 8 ounce serving sizes do you see? What I see is 12 and 16 ounces very common. Now we are hitting

20 and even 32 ounce drinks that people grab and guzzle down and pack on the pounds, not fully realizing they have been bamboozled by a large company offering what seems to be a good deal because it is a huge quantity. Marketers know that most people will not turn down a larger quantity for only a slightly higher price. They make a lot of sales and they make a few more pennies every time a consumer falls for this type of marketing. The worst thing out of all this super sizing and one-up marketing by large companies, as a nation we have totally lost touch with reality of a normal serving size. Even worse, if you have young kids and they see these huge portions, they are growing up not knowing any better, they will grow up thinking this is the norm when it is not the norm and these huge serving sizes are a huge factor why we are obese.

If you opened up a restaurant and served small, normal serving size portions of food and drink you would be out of business before you even got started. People would laugh at the small portion that you served on their plates. They would demand to have their plates filled to capacity and demand their super sized drinks with free refills, the bottomless bread basket, or the endless salad bar. If you tried to explain that you were serving normal portions that were healthy and good for their diets and that 8 ounces of soda was all you were bringing for the entire meal, I bet your customers would leave and never return and they would tell all their friends about your small portions and bad deal. So you can easily see why chain restaurants offer larger and larger and larger portions. It has the same effect, people talk and word gets around that restaurant x down the street is offering such huge portions you won't believe it.

I took a friend out for dinner and we ordered an appetizer to split, plus our dinners. When the appetizer arrived we could not believe the size of the plate and the quantity of food on the huge plate. We looked at each other in disbelief. There was enough food on the appetizer plate for both of us without the regular dinner. When all of our food came to the table there was easily enough to feed 4. We were being served way too much and we were eating way to many calories for the entire day at one sitting. I took another friend out to a new restaurant that just opened and I remember that the portions were plenty large and on top of that I remember the waitress bringing free refills on our drinks without us requesting them and before our drinks were empty. I thought to myself it was nice service but a total waste, as I said we were not even done with our first drink and here she was bringing us another 20 ounce drink that I had no need for. I took a few sips and the rest went down the drain. <u>What a waste I thought.</u> For other people I am sure they loved the free refill and the extra 20 ounce drink simply because it was free. An extra 20 ounce drink is a lot of calories on top of the huge portions. [I don't care if it was a diet drink either. If you are sucking down 20 or 30 ounces of a beverage at one meal it is way too much. I just don't see where these diet drinks are so great for your body or your health. Sure, a mildly foul tasting beverage with 0 calories and an artificial sweetener that we are not 100% sure just how bad it may be, I don't see diet beverages being advertised as the perfect food that your body has been dying for.] I feel we are getting way too many free, unwanted calories when we go out to eat that people can't shed later. This super size marketing approach has hit almost every food product we buy or order out and I see no sign of it stopping any time soon. As you observe new TV ads and new product packaging you will now see what I am talking about.

Another negative side effect is when we are cooking at home, we are so used to the huge portions of food we get in restaurants or at the convenient marts, it seems ludicrous when we are eating and drinking normal serving sizes at home or in our lunch packed at home. Personally, I buy a lot of individual serving size foods for my lunch instead of eating out everyday for lunch. This is when I started noticing the difference in serving sizes. I will give you some quick examples. I buy 100% pure oj in a six pack and they are 8 ounces, a single serving and the box looks tiny, but that is what I drink for lunch. [I remember when I was in school and we were served a little box of milk with our lunch.] Another one I love is the fruit cup or tiny individual serving sizes of applesauce. As I write this I am noticing my use of tiny and small as I describe a <u>normal serving size</u> and it is because, as I have mentioned, our 21st century one-up marketing distorted serving size. Even the packaging in the grocery stores reflect this to a certain degree. I think about the packaging of steaks, for example. 2 nice steaks for a couple to enjoy, weighing in at hefty 12 ounces each and in portion size with a steak you might get in a nice restaurant. Realistically, a nice 12 ounce boneless steak is plenty for 2 to enjoy. That is about 6 ounces each, and although it is half of what you would usually get out in a restaurant, it is 2 serving sizes of meat. A serving size of steak is about 3 ounces, so even with the small portion of splitting one steak you are still getting 2 servings at home. Depending on the cut of steak, your calories for a 6 ounce portion can range from about 300 to 400 calories for a small 6 ounce portion. Now as we have discussed, on a 2000 calorie diet you only have about 650 calories per meal so you can see just how little you can add to your dinner at home with the very small piece of steak before you are over budget for that meal. Just something to think about and put the huge restaurant portions into perspective.

#20 READING LABELS FOR CALORIES AND INGREDIENTS

I really think it is time for the people in this country to wake up and open their eyes. Almost everything we buy has a list of ingredients and calorie chart listed on the package. I think if most people started taking notice and reading the labels it just might be enough to change the way they eat and buy food and drink. We need to start moving away from foods that have an ingredients list a mile long with words we can't even pronounce and we need to start moving toward a more natural unprocessed diet (as in foods you buy fresh and cook on the stove). Once I started reading labels for calories and ingredients it completely changed my habits. The simple cure for me was looking at a label for my favorite corn chip and after seeing the long list of ingredients that were being slapped on a simple corn chip, I decided this food was not for me. There is plenty of danger in daily life already that I need not be adding to it by eating these types of foods on a daily basis. There is so much good healthy food for us to eat that we should not be bamboozled by fancy labels, marketing, or convenience to buy this over processed food with way too many mystery ingredients. Keep reading the labels on the bad food you eat until one day the lights go off and you tell yourself that I really don't need to be putting all these terrible, artificial ingredients in my body.

The same holds true for calories, saturated fat, and cholesterol on these labels. When I started taking notice I could not believe how many calories and fat you could stuff into junk food. I was simply shocked by some of the high calorie foods I was eating and not having a clue, these labels also give you a break down on saturated fat and cholesterol as a percentage based on a 2000 calorie daily intake. I hope you are shocked to find out how high some of these numbers are on the junk foods that we eat. I hope that if you see a label that says 40% saturated fat in one little package of junk food that you are about to eat, it gets your attention. On the other hand, what I discovered was in comparison how low in calories all the good food is vs. the junk food. I highly recommend you buy a small book on food values and calories. I was very surprised to see how low in calories fruits and vegetables were vs. the junk food. I was pleasantly surprised to see that you could eat meat and fish in small portions and not blow your calories for the day or die of a heart attack. If you flip through the book on calories in different foods, you will see how much of the good stuff you can eat and still maintain your weight or what adjustments you will have to make to lose weight. The book will cost approximately 5 dollars (most large book stores have these little pocket guides on food and calories) and in my opinion the information you discover inside is priceless. The last thing you need to be paying attention to is the serving size or number of servings per package. As with many prepackaged ready to eat foods of super size portions, they will contain 2 or 3 servings per package. You must pay attention to this. Just because you are buying a bag or a bottle of this or that, don't be fooled thinking it is a single serving. I am looking at a bottle (a monster 20 oz super size bottle) of juice right now and it says 110 calories per serving, carbs 10% and sugar value of 28g x 2.5 servings in this container!!! I will do the math for you. 275 calories, 25% of your total carbs for the day and a whopping 70g on the sugar. You must pay close attention to these labels and think about what you are about to eat or pour into your body. As I have said this isn't a get slim quick and easy program. It is a get slim and fit making small, daily adjustments over the long term for the rest of your life, but you must pay attention everyday, every meal.

#21 THINKING ABOUT THE CHILDREN

As I look around at the kids these days I am shocked to see little kids obese everywhere I go. I see lots of heavy kids and I mean of all ages, from 3 right through teens. As parents I feel it is your responsibility to get this handled before your children are burdened with obesity for the rest of their lives. Now I know full well when they hit their teens and start working and driving and getting on their own it becomes much harder to guide them, but there is no excuse that I want to hear when I see the little ones already obese!!! This is a serious problem that must be addressed and I feel the sooner in life the better. As far as I know an 8 year old cannot drive to the store and buy junk food and a 3 year old is not making his own prime rib dinner with all the trimmings yet and eating a 14 ounce monster portion of meat and a 5 year old should not be ordering like a wild man when dining out with his parents. I usually like the saying that we should lead by example, but in this instance that is what I see too much of. Huge parents with huge kids.

Another saying I like is you will do more for others than you will ever do for yourself and maybe you need to think about changing your own eating habits so you can help your kids and yourself at the same time. This overspending on food could be ruining your finances if you have a couple of kids and your food budget is out of control. The money savings is meaningless compared with the potential long term negative effects on their health, being picked on in school, and as an adult battling weight problems for the rest of their lives.

As a family, maybe it's time for a sit down and everyone pulling together for a major change in lifestyle, eating, shopping, snacking, and dining out habits. Maybe it's time for the parents to sit down and just rough out the food budget and just get an idea how much money you are throwing away on junk food per week x 52 and see how much this adds up to. There are about a thousand ways to get creative here with the family all involved and slim everyone down together. <u>This is a time to get creative and have fun in the process.</u> At minimum it's a time to realize that we have a problem and we need to address it before it gets completely out of control. M a n y sections of this course can be applied to the children (let them read it, too) but first you need to acknowledge that you have a problem and then make changes to correct the problem. I really feel for most kids it is the huge supply of junk food and soda that is lying around the house in every cupboard, pantry and freezer and with a minimum amount of effort they can be pigging out with the push of a button on the microwave or slapping a frozen item in the oven or chugging down another soda. To compound the problem there are very few chores to be done around the house anymore, which leads to a very inactive lifestyle and very few calories burned playing video games or watching TV all day long and constantly snacking. Bottom line here is, someone, as in an adult, is bringing this junk food into the house, or someone is not preparing balanced and nutritious meals and limiting the portions, or someone is allowing too much dining out with the super size portions. Each household must identify its problem areas and get them handled. This problem will not go away by itself. It only gets worse with time. As they get older and as adults they wonder why they are obese and wonder why they can't eat like pigs and lose weight or be normal or be healthy. Again, I feel the super size kids are a sign of our wealth in this country, being able to buy all the expensive junk food and being able to dine out on a regular basis and order with little or no restriction. I feel healthy and active little munchkins with a little parental control on food intake should have little or no weight problem and they certainly should not be labeled obese!!!

When I was growing up we lived in the country and I was very active and I loved being outside. There was always plenty to do, video games were not real big yet and snacking between meals was not a real issue. We ate good, solid, healthy meals and we only went out for dinner on special occasions. But times have changed drastically for kids and our society as a whole in the last 20 to 30 years and we must think about things differently and we must make positive changes in our lives. If you can't do it for yourself, maybe you can take a stand for your kids. Maybe it is time to take a good look in the mirror and maybe it is time you took a good look at your kids and see if you like what you see and if you are happy with your job as a parent. If you don't like what you see maybe this self evaluation will force you to make changes for everyone's sake. Our kids seem to be lacking parental involvement in many areas of their lives. Maybe starting with the food issue will open more doors for better communication in other areas of their lives, too.

The bottom line is we have to start somewhere and we have to take action or nothing changes............... I know most parents love their children more than anything in the world and they would never let anyone ever hurt them and they only want the very best for them. But letting your little ones eat themselves to obesity at a young age is no good and I feel it is the parent's responsibility to get this handled. Some say it takes a village to raise a child and to me that is the biggest bunch of socialist bullshit I have ever heard. It takes a mother and a father to raise a child. It takes a mother and a father to step up and take responsibility for their own children. I know there is the divorce issue and the kids being bounced from parent to parent with no one stepping up and taking responsibility for discipline and the kids rebelling and basically being out of control. You know what, that is a poor excuse in my book!!! I see way too many little kids in public completely out of control and the parents just looking on like, oh well, this is life in the 21st century. Don't blame your ex and don't blame society for your ill behaving kids. Stop blaming everyone else and start pointing the finger at yourself. Take responsibility!!!

I have seen the show where 6, 8 and 10 year old kids are running the household and the parents sit there like morons and seem to not have a clue how to manage an 8 year old. Personally I think it's pathetic!!! I don't care how much or how little money you make in your career and how big of a success you think you are. If your kids are out

Robert K. Christiansen

of control and your relationships suck, you are not a success...............
The last time I knew it didn't cost a nickel to sit down and talk with
your kids or better yet listen to them and see what they have to say
and listen to them as they pour their feelings/concerns out to you. <u>A
little communication can make all the difference and I am not talking
about food and weight alone here either. Good communication can
make a huge difference in your kid's entire life.</u>

#22 BREAKING THE CYCLE

There comes a time in a person's life or even in a culture or a nation when something major changes and things are never the same (some call them paradigm shifts). I could cite many examples but I feel you get the picture. A person must get to a point in their lives when they say enough is enough and adjust their course.............. It seems we have been sucked into a way of life in this country over the last 20 to 30 years that really doesn't suit many of us and I think it's time we all took a hard look at all major areas of our lives. I know we are focusing on the battle of the bulge in this course, but breaking the cycle can be applied to many parts of our lives. It is time to take a stand, it is time for a change. We need to get some control in our lives and stop being led around by ads on the TV and radio for the next quick fix. It seems like the majority of ads I see on TV are for either drugs to make you feel better or cure some ailment you may or may not have (but ask your doctor if this drug might be right for you) or for exercise equipment or the new weight loss miracle pill the world has been waiting for. Some of the ads are so ridiculous I can't believe anyone could be so <u>stupid</u> to fall for it. Being an intelligent person you must ask yourself the same simple common sense question I did. If all these diet pills and exercise products we are bombarded with in ads on a daily basis worked, why is obesity completely out of control in our country? It is time for you to stop being super sized by big business and it is time you took a stand, it is time you told yourself this old way of life is not for me anymore. It is time to break the cycle and it starts with you today..............

#23 A CHAT WITH MY BROTHER

My bro is not a rocket scientist nor is he a doctor, but we did have an interesting conversation one day as I talked about this course (something interesting I heard on TV and something interesting he had been reading about). What I heard on TV was a shocking statistic that about 10% of the population in NYC had sugar diabetes, and I wondered if it had a lot to do with the fact that those people live in tall buildings and probably don't have much to do in an apartment and probably are not as active as they should be and probably overweight. We talked about the obesity problem in this country and people seeming to not have a clue. Then he mentioned something that I found interesting. He mentioned a book he was reading that talked about obesity and the body storing excessive consumed sugar as fat (especially in the mid section), and as you look around or in the mirror and see people bulging in the mid section that is a lot of stored fat/sugar on the body. What he said made sense to me. Again, we are not doctors, but in a nutshell the pancreas plays its part with the insulin in the bloodstream in a healthy person's body, but with all this excess sugar/fat stored on an overweight (being obese is even worse) person's body the pancreas goes on the fritz or shuts down and basically says, if you're going to keep pouring all that excessive sugar into me, I am going on strike, and the kidneys say they will join me next, because when I go on strike the kidneys get overworked (the kidneys filter the waste from the blood) and they throw the towel in, too, or they may shut down completely.

<u>HELLO!!! ANYONE</u> <u>LISTENING UP THERE?</u> Now, I know some people are born with sugar diabetes, but recently it is turning into a huge non hereditary problem, like bang, out of nowhere. As I mentioned we are not doctors, but could it be this simple? Could all the excess sugar, fat, preservatives, cholesterol, salt, and calories that we consume that turns us into porkers be causing all kinds of problems within our bodies? Something to think about before you pig out again. Maybe it is our bodies trying to communicate with us again in the only way it knows how? Stop, you are killing us!!! Give this some thought.............. I am sure if you go online you can get the exact function of every cell in the human body so you can come to your own scientific conclusion and maybe give you a better understanding of just how thin the balance beam we walk on a daily basis with our bodies is between being healthy and happy and killing ourselves prematurely.

#24 YOU DIDN'T GET FAT OVERNIGHT AND YOU'RE NOT GOING TO GET SLIM OVERNIGHT

You didn't get fat overnight and you are not going to get slim overnight.

Now, what part of this don't you understand? I know it seems you can look at a piece of cake or eat 2 donuts or sit down to a fancy meal and it seems like you gain 2 pounds, bam, just like that. Fact is you have to eat about 3500 calories to gain one pound. Chances are you are not eating 7000 extra calories in one day and gaining 2 pounds overnight. I will give you that at times the weight does seem to jump on without you knowing it and it comes off tougher than removing super glue, but bottom line is, you didn't gain it overnight and you are not going to lose it overnight. <u>You must understand this people!!!</u>

It kills me when I see all the new tricky ads on TV for all these different pills that guarantee to melt the fat off your body overnight. I love the drama, "Oh, it's not your fault you are fat"............... (<u>well who the hell's fault is it then?!!!</u>) In my daily travels I don't see anyone being force fed, so take responsibility. It is your fault. I know some people have medical conditions and there is no hope for them, but my point is, I believe 99% of the healthy people in this country are capable of maintaining a comfortable and healthy weight if they would just wake up, take responsibility, and make some minor adjustments in their lives. Our blame everybody else for our problems mentality must stop in this country. <u>I am tired of people not taking responsibility!!!</u> In my opinion, any ad that states immediate results, easy results, while you still stuff your face is a flat out rip off. Are we really that stupid in this country? Are people that easily misled? Are we really that desperate for the quick fix that we are willing to spend a lot of money for a false hope sold by a glamorous movie star that we know in our hearts will not work? In this fast paced world that we live in we want immediate results with no effort on our part. We want everything done for us and we want it done now. Well, I am here to break some bad news to you. It is your fault you are fat!!! Unless you are a total loser or a total moron, don't waste your money on these quack remedies. Furthermore, if one of these miracle pills actually worked, wouldn't everyone be slim and happy with their weight?

Look, the numbers don't lie. I don't know the exact percentage that are considered overweight or obese (and it is constantly on the rise/change) but it is staggeringly high. Moreover, wouldn't a caring friend have told you by now which miracle pill to buy to solve all your problems? OK professor Bert, yep, you can eat like a pig and take this magic pill and you will be slim as a movie star in 2 weeks. Not!!! (I have sprinkled this course with a little humor here and there.) Wouldn't we have one company that figured it out and had the entire market and that company would be worth billions of dollars? If one of these get slim quick advertisements actually produced the said results, why are there 20 different companies selling all these quack remedies and people still so overweight in this country? I am looking for an answer folks, I can't hear youuuuuuuuuuuuuu!!! Common sense would have to whisper in your ear at this point and say, "Because these quack remedies simply do not work long term." There is no quick fix. (good answer grasshopper)

A good friend of mine once said, "There is nothing common about common sense." I hope you think about this quote. OK, I will cut these fast cure people a tiny bit of slack here. Maybe they work for a temporary few pounds of weight loss for a handful of people, but I do not see them having any effect on the number of fat people (long term) in this country, the number just seems to have grown out of control over the last 20 years. Have we not seen an explosion of quack remedies and exercise equipment being sold, chasing the trend? People have spent billions of dollars on these attractively advertised products with little or no results. I hope you spend some time thinking about this and who really made out? Funny, even the corporations selling these products got fat. lol

#25 ADJUSTING FOR A
LIFETIME OF SUCCESS

Let's get to the meat of this chapter. In my opinion there is no overnight success. The pills, the powders, the prepackaged food, the exercise equipment, has not had the desired results that we have been promised. The proof again is in the staggering number of fat people. The numbers don't lie. In my opinion the simple reason is people are not getting to the root of the problem and B, people do not stick with the changes. <u>The root of the problem is people are simply eating too many calories/food and not burning enough of it off on a daily basis.</u> I wish it was more scientific but that's it in a nutshell. That's the root of the problem that no one seems to be talking about, probably because it is not very scientific and probably because they aren't going to make billions of dollars profit telling people it is as simple as this..............

There was a line in a movie and the actor said, "You can't handle the truth." I love that line and I think it's time we started handling the truth instead of sugar coating everything in this country. We already have way too much sugar in our diet as it is.............. Over a period of time we are gaining weight one pound at a time until we are fat or obese. We don't need the pills if we get to the root of the problem and that again is as simple as eating what is necessary to live. The prepackaged food deals are no deal. Few will stick with those programs for the rest of their lives. I have seen those boxes of food first hand (I was visiting someone who had just purchased a meal plan from a TV ad and we were kicking the box around in disbelief and joking about the actual product/garbage received). I will give them credit for great marketing and awesome camera work but I wondered what happened to the delicious looking food from the TV ad. Personally, I would never eat one thing that was in that box and I don't even think most people would feed it to their pets. What an eye opener that was for me. Bottom line, it was expensive, the food looked disgusting, and it came in an unrefrigerated box so you can imagine the preservatives. The only one that made out was the big fat corporation!!! So if you haven't tried that plan yet my advice is save your coin...............

Weight loss equipment looks great, appears to work on these great looking slim models, is very expensive, and again has not had much of an affect on our fat society. Gyms are in almost every town and weight loss equipment can be bought everywhere. But I feel the problem lies in the fact that people do not stick with it for the long term. Personally, I tried working out. I bought weights and other things and it was great for the first couple of weeks, but I really had to force myself to do it. After a month the weights went into the closet and are still sitting there to this day and I never touched them again. Wasted money, no result. My favorite target here is the treadmill, a very expensive machine that everyone thinks is the magic bullet. Walk on it while they watch TV or have a snack and boom, I will be fit for life. It seems everyone has a treadmill at their house but they are using it for a hat rack. Now they have to be the most expensive hat racks I have ever seen in my life. Or you see them at a yard sale for 10 cents on the dollar waiting for another sucker to take it off their hands. Don't get me wrong here, if you like working out and that is your approach and you love doing it and you plan on doing it for the rest of your life, then you have found your key to success. Stick with it and you are set for life.

My point here is you must find something that works for you for the long haul. Adjusting for a lifetime is the key here. I know we took a round about way to get here but the bottom line to this section is getting over the fact that there are no quick fixes and any changes you make in your lifestyle and eating habits must be adhered to for the rest of your life. <u>This is a new way of life, thinking about everything that enters your mouth for the rest of your life.</u> Until you come to terms with this fact, I feel most will struggle with their weight throughout their life. The scary thing is eating an extra 500 calories per week (that is only an extra 70 unnecessary calories per day) x 52 weeks in a year gone unchecked for 5 years and you have porked on a whopping 37 pounds!!! 1000 extra unnecessary calories per week unchecked for 5 years and you could easily pack on 75 pounds!!! That is scary and I hope it gets your attention. I have seen women in wedding pictures a skinny/sexy size 5 and 5 years later a disgusting size 16 and it's like, "Who is that hottie in those wedding pics?", and after you realize you just stuck your foot in your mouth so far that there is no hope for a save you have to say to yourself, "Well, she is not recognizable from her wedding pictures just 5 years ago." Both men and women seem to fall into the marriage trap, getting comfortable and gaining lots of weight in 5 years. As they say, time flies and 5 years later you have gained 4 dress sizes or added 4 inches to the waist size of your jeans and you wake up one day totally disgusted with your body and your looks. On the flip side of the coin you can take this simple process and reverse the pounds right off too. The choice is yours. The key is consistency and a new lifestyle that you continue for the rest of your life, every minute of every day.

#26 TAKE A GOOD LOOK
AROUND AT SOCIETY

Recently I have been taking a good look around when I am out and about and I am stunned how fat, men, women and children are!!! I am not talking about people that are 10 pounds overweight either. I am talking about everywhere I look seeing people 50 or 100 pounds overweight!!! Little kids busting out of their clothes and waddling around their huge parents. Men that are so fat in the mid section that I wonder where they buy their pants, and women so fat, wearing stretch pants because nothing else fits!!! In my opinion, once you start wearing sweat pants or stretch pants because regular clothes are not comfortable, you lost the battle of the bulge!!! This is a very important point that you better get. I gauge my weight by how my clothes fit, I don't even have a scale in my house. Again, I only own the same size jeans, size 32-32 (keep in mind that I have been wearing the same size jeans for about 20 years), so everyday I am reminded all day long how I am doing with my diet according to how my jeans fit.

If you own different size clothes, I am going to recommend you start sorting through your clothes and focus on the size that you want to wear and is comfortable. The larger sizes have to go if you ever want to lose weight and when you hit your target weight you must have only one size that you buy and wear. My opinion is, if you weigh yourself in the AM and you know it is too much it is not powerful enough for you to think before you shove something in your mouth. But if your clothes are too tight all day long and not comfortable, you will think twice before stuffing your face with poison food. This may be one of the most important things I ever tell you and I hope you understand this. I will say it again about the stretchy pants. If you are serious about adjusting your weight and maintaining your weight, the stretchy pants must go!!! Having the larger sizes or stretchy pants in your closet tells me you are not committed. Throwing them in the garbage today is a major step in the right direction. Now you are committed. (I will give you a cute analogy about the difference between being involved and being committed. When you sit down to have breakfast this weekend and it is consisting of ham and eggs, the chicken was involved but the pig was committed...............) It is a clear sign you can never go back. It sends a clear message to yourself that you have had enough and it is time to get serious!!! The act of sorting through your clothes, trying them on, and tossing some in the garbage is a major step that must be taken. Now, failure is not an option, because you will have nothing to wear...............

Let's think about something here. We are all born of similar size. When we are kids we really don't know any better. But what the hell happened when you were a teen or twenties or thirties??? How did you go from a slim kid to a huge adult? Who bought the next size larger clothes and slipped them in your closet when you were busting out of the size you were wearing? (Another sign of our wealth in this country, being able to toss out our clothes because we can't fit in them anymore and buying a new wardrobe of larger sizes. That is a lot of money wasted, a lot of money (ladies).) I really feel everyone must ask themselves. How did I go from a size 7 to a size 14? How did I go from size 30 jeans to size 40? My opinion is that when your clothes didn't fit comfortable, instead of getting to the root of the problem, you just went out and bought the next size and the next size and the next size, until one day you looked in the mirror and didn't recognize the person looking back. Now, how about if we just reverse the process, starting today, throwing out all the loose, fat day clothes and start buying tighter, smaller sizes until we reach our comfortable/healthy/happy size? Another important point here, this did not happen overnight, getting larger and buying larger clothes and slimming down is not going to happen overnight either. This section might be the most powerful part of this course!!!

I want you to start observing people when you are out and about. Just look at the number of people that are huge and ask yourself silently, do I want to look like that? Is that the type of person I want to be? Ask yourself if you think that that person is miserable inside. These few questions and quick observations could change your life forever.

(another point I want to throw in) I feel our bodies undergo major change every 10 years. As we get older we tend to slow down, our bodies don't burn the calories like they used to and we are not as active. So what worked in our 30's is not necessarily going to work when we reach our 40's or 50's. When we retire and our whole life goes through a major change what worked for us earlier in life is not guaranteed to work at this point in our lives. The bottom line here is we need to keep fine tuning our eating habits as we age, we need to make adjustments as we age to keep our weight in check. When you start seeing what worked 10 years ago not working anymore, it is one of those ahhhhhhhhh moments in life. And you can either fine tune your eating, make adjustments in your lifestyle, or gain weight. Now that I have made you aware of this fact you will know how to handle it when it hits your life.

I will tell you a little personal story here. I didn't always have the weight game figured out either. When I was in my early thirties I went through some major changes in career and relationships and found myself falling into the (buy) larger jeans size syndrome. I spent about the last 10 years wearing 32-32 jeans say from age 22 to 32, then I found myself in a new town with a new job and a new girlfriend and lifestyle. (In addition, I was going through the 10 year change in my body, too, which I was not aware of at the time and didn't really figure this variable into my problem.) I was busting out of my 32-32 jeans for the first time and I didn't know what to do. I tried working out, new diets and so on with poor results, so I fell into the simple fix/trap that I feel most people fall into and get in trouble and basically lose the battle of the bulge. It was to buy (large) size 33 (waist) 32 jeans. I was literally busting out of my 32 waist to the point of not being able to comfortably button them. Now, the waist fit good on the larger size, but the legs were baggy and I did not like the way I looked or the way I felt about myself. (This is why I say that people that are obese, the majority, cannot feel good about themselves. I was only about 10 pounds over where I wanted to be and I was totally disgusted with myself.) I knew I had to figure something out, I knew I had to discover something.

What I discovered personally was that willpower, exercise, pills, drinks, and crash diets were not for me and they were not working. I wore my larger jeans a couple days a week and had to deal with busting out of my 32-32 jeans until I lost enough weight (figured things out) so they were comfortable again. To my amazement after about a month of being disgusted 5 days a week in my tight jeans with the button opened and being disgusted with myself when I wore my larger fatty jeans I started eating a little different. I started eating a little less each meal and each day. I also started eating more nutritious foods and less junk food and less fast food, especially when I was wearing my tight jeans. The tight jeans were a constant reminder to me all day long that I was overweight and not happy with it and it made me uncomfortable enough to control what I ate during the day. The tight jeans were powerful enough to make me stop eating the junk food, and the tight jeans were powerful enough to make me drive past the fast food joints to avoid the poison calories. The tight jeans were a constant reminder to me all day long that I needed to change my ways. (As I said, weighing yourself on a scale in the am is not powerful enough for most people to take control of their food intake.) By shoving a little less food in my mouth each day and thinking about what I was shoving in my mouth, I could button my 32 jeans again after about a month. They were still tight, but I could button them. After about 3 months of making small adjustments everyday in the right direction, I noticed on the days I wore my 33 waist jeans that they were falling off my ass if I had my hands in my pockets and pushing down a little. I also noticed my 32-32 jeans were very comfortable again. On that day I tossed my 33 fat jeans out and never bought another pair or even thought about it.

On the day I tossed the fatty jeans out it was a very good feeling. It was a very powerful feeling to be in control. It was very powerful knowing that I had won the battle on my own and without the help of an organization or without having to have had my hand held by a sponsor or a coach or the use of a magic pill. There is no better feeling in the world like figuring something out on your own and getting things handled. Moreover, you can apply this take action, get it done approach to many areas of your life. If I didn't get to the root of the problem and figure things out and take action, over the years I would have probably grown into an obese slob.

Another 10 years have passed since that major change/discovery in my life and I am still wearing my 32-32 jeans and I can't see ever buying a different size for the rest of my life. I still don't have a scale in my house either.

#27 TAKING ACTION

They say that knowledge is power............... and I say bullshit. You can be the smartest, most informed person on earth and if you don't take action and apply your knowledge it will be of no use to you. A wise man once said, "Many receive advice, but only the wise benefit from it." I feel 100% that you have to get to a point in your life where you have had enough. Whether it be weight loss, quitting smoking, a bad job or a bad relationship or whatever, but I do feel you have to get to a point where you just say that's it. You get pissed at yourself, you slam your hands on the table and say that's it!!! I hope you are at that point in your life with your weight and overall well-being and that is the reason for ordering this course.

Furthermore, I hope you are ready to take massive action and change your old ways. If you have read this material thoroughly (I highly recommend you read it several times and even reference it in the future), I feel that most healthy people can change their lives forever and really never be burdened with a weight problem the rest of their lives. Successful people take action!!! Informed successful people lead the pack in almost every area of life. The most important thing I can tell you here is you have the knowledge now to change, and it is up to you to take action. The greatest thing here is that it is up to you and no one else!!! Think about this............... So many areas of our lives are so tied to other people. I feel it is hard to make positive change in so many other areas of our lives because it involves so many other people and it is very hard to move others in the same direction we want to go. You can't control the weather for a special outdoor event. If it rains and ruins your day the weather is completely out of your control. The greatest thing about taking action and adjusting your weight for a lifetime is that it is only up to you and no one can get in your way. There is no one to blame except yourself. I don't know of one person on earth that is force fed food............... You must think about this until you understand it. It can and will change your life. Furthermore, once you gain control over food and get down to your comfortable weight, <u>taking action, taking responsibility, and stop blaming everyone else for your problems,</u> you can start applying this success to many other areas of your life!!! The greatest feeling will be when you start taking action and you start seeing results. When you gain control and you feel it inside, this will be one of the most powerful feelings you will ever experience. I encourage you to make positive change throughout your life, feel the power of positive change, feel the rush of taking action. <u>Just imagine how great every aspect of your life could be if you were in control 100% instead of being out of control.</u> I firmly believe people are fat pigs because they have little or no control. What kind of person do you want to be from today forward??? Just look around you everywhere you go. When you see a fat person it is pretty safe to assume they have 0 self control, 0 discipline and I bet they are miserable inside. Now, ask yourself silently, do I want to look like that or do I want to be in control of my life? This little observation and self test can change your way of thinking and way of life and put you in control.

[a little story] I remember one of my friends that quit smoking cold turkey after maybe 20 years of smoking cigs. One day he quit and never smoked another cig. I thought to myself, if he can do that he can accomplish anything he ever wanted to put his mind to. I never figured out how he did it, but I think he just got to a point and said no more!!! Took action, stopped smoking and never looked back.............................

#28 LOW STANDARDS

This may be a little bitch session on my part but I think maybe some will relate to it, some may be humored by it, and some may really appreciate it if they just stop and think about it. It seems to me that in the last 20 to 30 years we have really lowered our standards in this country to the basement level. From food, to service, to general products we buy on a daily basis imported from all over the world. It seems we can't buy anything made in the U. S. anymore. Focusing on the food for now (the big picture later) it seems we as consumers only buy because we are either getting the lowest price or the best deal as in huge portions. <u>The lowest price buying has driven the quality out of every part of our lives.</u> As I said I love to cook, and don't get me wrong, I also enjoy a good meal out, too. Recently I have noticed while dining out the low quality of food being served and even a lower level of service. In an effort to supply a dinner at the lowest possible price to stay competitive with the explosion of chain restaurants on every corner fighting for the consumers' dollars and the ever shrinking pie that just keeps getting sliced thinner due to all the competition, the standards of quality food and service have been lowered to the basement. It's shocking to me to see all the small shop owners disappearing one by one, slowly but surely being steamrolled by the guaranteed lowest price, lowest quality chains, and this is not only in the restaurant business. If you take a good look around it is in almost every area of our lives. High quality products/high quality service being replaced with low quality offered at a low price.

Recently I have noticed the quality of food and service going downhill at 3 restaurants (small family operations) that I used to go to on occasion, and it's really sad to see things slipping away. As the consumer lowers their standards (and has the cheapest only mentality, we are all going to suffer) the shop owners must cut costs in an effort to stay competitive and compete on price alone because nobody appreciates high quality at a reasonable price anymore. <u>As we accept the lower standards we are accepting a lower quality of life.</u> Going out for a nice relaxing dinner is a treat for me, but when I see and taste the low quality of food that I am being served and a waitress that only seems to be there to see how much of a tip she can get out of each table and really doesn't give a flying ..... about her level of service or professionalism she is providing, I am turned off on the whole experience. I am almost shocked when I observe on a daily basis almost everywhere I go and see how low we have lowered our standards in this country.

I remember telling a friend about a dining experience I had at a restaurant we both went to and I simply told her that the food I was served was not up to my standards anymore and I would not be going there for a long time or until they changed things around. She said she had not been very satisfied either lately with the food and pretty much had the same feelings I did about this 2 generation establishment. Due to the lower standards, we have both checked this restaurant off our list and I have been going there for the last 15 years!!! Another place that I used to go to that had a pretty good reputation for quality food and good service I recently found has been bitten by the low quality, low price bug, too. As I walked into the restaurant I noticed a few things that seemed a little odd. The first minor thing was some misspelled words on the special board and I kinda chuckled and blew it off to some new help. The second thing I noticed, usually this place was hopping with a bustling dinner crowd and I was almost shocked when I saw how few people were there eating. When I received my dinner it all came together for me, a huge portion of low quality food. This place used to be known for high quality tasty meals with a lot of things being made in house with the best ingredients. When I started eating my dinner the first bites told the whole story. My food was of the lowest quality and to boot it was bordering on being served cold. I picked through about 30% of my meal and pushed it away. I sat there thinking, "Boy, this place has lowered its standards to the basement and it's showing by the lack of customers." It was showing by the fact that 2 or 3 waitresses were standing around complaining about no business and nothing to do. When my waitress asked if I wanted a box to package my huge remaining portion of food, I said no, that I was full. I thought to myself even the local semi wild cats near my house would probably not even eat it. Hell, they have standards too and I must say they are pretty high. They are used to my premium scraps that they are treated to on occasion and I would not want to disappoint them or be embarrassed serving them the low quality of food that I was served at that restaurant.

I have hit upon the little guy trying to compete with the corporate giants in the restaurant business and I think it is time we actually looked at the low quality of food that we accept as consumers at our favorite chain restaurant. The more I dine out the less I enjoy the whole experience. I honestly feel the large chains buy the lower or lowest quality food they can find so they can offer huge portions at a reasonable price to draw in customers. Moreover, the reasonable price usually turns into a hefty bill by the time we are done. When I dine out there are very few things I order. I know most selections on most menus are made in a factory, flash frozen, shipped to the restaurant and microwaved to a perfect glow just before serving. I am very disappointed that we have lowered our standards to accept this type of low quality food and pay a good price for it and wait on line for an hour and consider this a good experience. A wise neighbor once said, "If you want good food, stay home and cook." As I see the low level of quality and service we accept at a restaurant I am very disappointed. You would think if one was going to pack on 2000 calories eating a big dinner out, the food should be exquisite. The total experience wonderful. You would think if one was going to pay a hefty total price for dinner out the service should be top notch, and anything short of top notch would not be acceptable. (As consumers we should reward low quality products and service providers with a statement and that statement would be that we will be back when you raise the standards. In 6 months this establishment will have raised its standards or be out of business. Either way the consumer wins and society as a whole wins, too.)

If you don't know what exquisite food should taste like I feel sorry for you and highly recommend you watch some cooking shows or take cooking classes. At minimum, get a good cookbook and start trying to cook. If a real chef tasted most items on a chain restaurant's menu and then saw how they were prepared, I think most dishes would be thrown in the garbage and the kitchen staff ordered to prepare the dish properly or be fired immediately. Oops, I almost forgot, chain restaurants don't hire professionally trained chefs, they can't afford to (furthermore, any chef worth his salt would walk off the job in the first hour after looking at the low quality and prepackaged garbage he would be required to cook). They hire microwavers (can you feel the radar love???), deep fry station managers, grill masters (yea right), salad fluffers, defrost, sauce and burn under the broiler specialists.

[a little story] I remember a new steak house that opened in town, so I took a friend to try it out and it sure had all the glitz and glitter we have come to expect in a new chain. The steaks were proudly displayed as we walked in and you could even pick the one you wanted. The grill master would cook it to perfection and serve you the best steak you have ever eaten. I was sold right out of the gate, steak is what I was getting. I picked my steak out and then I observed (perhaps to steal a secret or two from the master). The first thing I noticed that slightly turned me off was that the grill master looked like he was still drunk from the evening before. Being front and center for all to see he took no pride in his appearance and I guess the restaurant didn't either or was to afraid to tell him.? I cut him some slack on his outward appearance and paid more attention to his technique in preparing me a world class steak. This was, after all, a steak house. I watched as he took the steak that I personally selected and literally covered it in seasoning salt and slapped it on the fire. At this point I was no longer impressed with the glitz and glitter of the new steak house, so I took my seat and hoped for a miracle, as I did not like what I saw. As I cut into my steak, my thoughts about this whole deal were confirmed. It was absolutely the worst steak that I have ever cut into. It was tough and it was as salty as the deep blue sea. If I prepared a steak that bad at home I would have treated the local kitty cats to a treat and went hungry that evening as I figured out what went so terribly wrong. If I prepared a steak that bad for friends or family I would be embarrassed. Needless to say, I have rewarded that restaurant with no more of my hard earned dollars. They got the glitz and glitter right but in my opinion they weren't backing it up with a quality steak. I think if we took the glitz and glitter out of these chain restaurants and graded them based on the quality of the food and service, I believe most would quietly disappear like a sand castle as high tide comes in. As the giant chain stores take over with the lowest price, lowest level of service, and the lowest quality guarantees, I hope we will all be happy. As we lower our standards to basement levels that is what we are going to get, <u>low quality</u> at low prices. This trend is not limited to restaurants, either. This low, low, lowwwwwwwww price mentality will affect every area of our lives. Low quality food in huge portions is adding to our obesity problem. Low quality imported products in discount stores that fail after the second use may break our economy!!! I hope at minimum, a few people will take a stand with me and raise your standards and not accept such low quality as the norm, be it dining out or buying imported junk from discount stores. One of the best ways to improve the quality of your life (in all areas!!!) is <u>raise your standards!!!</u>

#29 CHANGING YOUR IDENTITY

Until you change your identity, I feel most people will never win the battle of the bulge. Until you change who you are on the inside, and how you think about yourself, and how you internally communicate with yourself, I don't think the outside will change for the long term. Personally, I feel our strength is within. I see way too many people looking for strength from outside themselves or from belonging to groups or hand holding. I feel the more we look outside of ourselves for strength the weaker we become. Discover your inner strengths, develop inner strength. No one can take it away, and you can use it in many areas of your life!!!

[a little story] The story of the frog and the scorpion has been told many times in an attempt to demonstrate identity and it is one of my favorites. One day a scorpion wanted to cross a stream. The scorpion being unable to swim approached a frog and asked if he would let him ride on his back. The frog told the scorpion, "No, because if we get half way across and you decide to sting me I will die." The scorpion replied, "Mr. frog I would not do that because if I sting you I will die too, that would be silly............." After a little more persuading, the frog agreed, and the scorpion got on the frog's back and they started to swim across the stream. Half way across the stream (sure enough) the scorpion stings the frog!!! The frog cannot believe it!!! The frog screams out, "Why did you do that, why did you sting me!!!? Now we are both going to die!!!" The scorpion said, "Because I am a scorpion and that is what scorpions do, they sting frogs.............." I love that story and I think it is a great example of identity: who we are, how we communicate to ourselves, and why we do what we do.

Until the little voices in your head start communicating internally (identity change) that I am slim, healthy, and happy, I don't fall for quick fixes or quack remedies, I am not a consumer of junk food or poison food, I am no longer an undisciplined person that eats monster portions, I only eat the amount of food I need to stay healthy and remain slim because that's how slim people think, and this is my new identity - most people will struggle with our modern day battle of the bulge their whole lives. The pills and the exercise equipment may be a temporary fix but I think they are not working in the long term because we are not changing our identity.

When a non smoker walks past a display of cigarettes, they don't stop and look over the selection, they keep right on walking because they have no need for cigarettes because they are non smokers. A non drinker walks right past the beer cooler with no problem because they are a non drinker. A vegetarian walks right past the meat counter because they don't eat meat. If you have ever known a vegetarian that was doing it on willpower alone, you probably see them slipping here and there and most that I have seen trying to do it on will power alone don't seem to stick with being a vegetarian over the long haul. On the other hand if you know a vegetarian and it is their identity that they are a vegetarian, they can go their whole life and never backslide and never wrestle with not eating meat. This is not willpower, this is identity!!!

Willpower is weak, identity is strong. This is very important and you must understand this part and you must think about things in your own life that you can compare the above situations with. This may be another good place to get out paper and pen and do a little soul searching. Divide the paper into 3 columns. At the top of each column write: [1st column] Things you would never, ever consider doing [2nd column] Areas where you waver [3rd column] Areas in your life where you are weak (bad habits that must be broken) and need immediate change. I highly recommend you do this exercise and this is something that can be done for the rest of your life. Every so often you can redo this exercise. Just think how great a life we could all live if we kept fine tuning our identity and replacing bad habits with positive identity change. Our entire planet could benefit from this!!!

[another interesting story] I recently heard some facts about people that win a large amount of money in the lottery. I guess your chances of winning big in the lottery are about 1 in a million, so this may be another area where you might want to save your coin. Anyway, what I found interesting was the fact that most people that won a lot of money in the lottery filed for bankruptcy about 5 years after winning (many got divorced, too). I was very surprised/shocked when I heard this. The only reason I add this story is because I feel it has a lot to do with identity. The only sense I can make of a person that wins big and then blows it all and more, to the point of having to file for bankruptcy is they did not change who they were. It was probably a great fun ride/party for a few years but I feel the old voices in their head, the old identity guided their bad decisions to get back to the old way of life, basically the old comfort zone that they were used to operating in. I think everyone must think about their identity (who we are and how do we communicate with ourselves, what are those little voices in our heads saying) and how it effects all areas of our lives.

In closing, I hope you enjoyed the material and I hope I opened your eyes. Furthermore, I hope you will use the knowledge and take action and change your entire life for the better and <u>live well and long.</u> In my opening, I stated that I wanted to be president to help people and make a positive change in our society. Perhaps this will be my contribution to society. I would like to be remembered as the one man that opened America's eyes and slimmed-er down. If that is one person at a time I truly hope it starts today with you. Many paradigm shifts start with one person and a great idea. Take action and join me today.............................

"EAT WELL, LOVE WELL AND LIVE WELL"

ROBERT K. CHRISTIANSEN

TIOGA TRADING, LLC.
World wide distributors of innovative products

BONUS PAGES

SUCCESS BY
ROBERT K. CHRISTIANSEN

#1 Know exactly what you want

#2 Find the right mate
   A) Be in love, make a happy home and live in peace.

#3 The right career
   A) Discover what you love doing and what you are good at.
   B) You will be successful doing what you love and you will be happy doing what you are good at.

#4 Goals
   A) Write down your goals and dreams without limits.
   B) Do you have what it takes to achieve your goals?
   C) Are you willing to put in the hours and pay the price to achieve your goals?
   D) How bad do you want to achieve your goals?
   E) Do you need to seek out a mentor?

#5 Make a plan
   A) Make a simple outline.

B) What steps need to be taken?
C) Take immediate action on your plan.
D) If your plan is not working, stop!!! Make a new plan.

"As you see yourself - you will become."
"As you think you deserve - you will receive."

#6 Know your desired outcome
   A) What are you trying to accomplish?
   B) What are the problems?
   C) What are the solutions?
   D) If your approach is not working, change it immediately.
   E) When you hit a wall, stop. Stop trying to climb a wall covered in grease. Take a break and walk around the wall.

#7 Make an agenda everyday
   A) What do I need to do today?
   B) Who do I need to call today?
   C) Who do I need to go see today?
   D) Your success depends on you, make no excuses.

#8 Work with the right people
   A) Get the right people on the ship.
   B) Get the right people in the right position.
   C) If an individual is not working out, fire them immediately. If a company is not producing the promised results, stop working with them immediately. Learn from your mistakes and press on wiser and stronger.
   D) 50% of the people that you work with will be losers, sort them out quickly!!!

#9 The journey
   A) Lifes journey will have many steps and many twists and turns. Lifes puzzle has many pieces, some bitter, some sweet.

B) Be thankful for what you have and where you are at today.
C) Be excited where you are going tomorrow.
D) Keep the big picture in mind and enjoy every step it takes to get there.
E) Enjoy today!!!

"The road that you are on - is it taking you where you want to be?"

#10 Network with successful people
    A) Form a mastermind group and have brainstorming sessions.
    B) Partner with successful people.
    C) What are they doing that makes them successful?

#11 The most successful people in your area
    A) What business are they in?
    B) Talk with them, ask how they became successful.
    C) Success leaves clues.

#12 List your strengths and weaknesses
    A) Focus on your strengths and hone your best skills.
    B) Hire the very best people to handle everything else and watch them closely.

#13 Know the money
    A) How much money do you net annually?
    B) What are your annual expenses? (Do a budget every year)
    C) What percentage of your income do you have left after all expenses?
    D) How do you start making more money today?
    E) How much are you saving and investing?
    F) Do an annual financial statement so you know how much you are worth.

G) Financially, where will you be in 1 year, 5 years, 10 years?
H) What is your financial plan for retirement?
I) At what age do you want to retire? How will you live?
J) Does your income need to increase for you to be more comfortable and have a solid financial future? What changes need to be made?
K) What can you do, starting today, to change your financial plan?
L) Where are you throwing money away?

"Until you reach beyond what you have already mastered - you will never be more than what you already are."

#14 Everything in moderation
A) Work, vacation and sex.
B) Food and drink. (No smoking and no drugs)
C) Risk, loans, credit.

#15 Keep educating and improving yourself
A) Read books and listen to audio programs.
B) Associate with intelligent and successful people.
C) Buy an unabridged dictionary and improve your vocabulary.

#16 Understand a few things before you start
A) There will be obstacles, disappointments and failures. These are only tests to see how wise you are, how resilient you are, how tough you are and how creative you are.
B) "The harder the fight, the sweeter the victory."
C) The ladder of success has many steps. Take a break, take a vacation, take a look through another eyes, take a new path, talk to a trusted friend, but never, ever, quit!!! Only the wise and determined will ever experience success. And they don't give big trophies for little effort.

D) The battle that doesn't kill you will make you wiser, stronger and more determined. Walk with wise men. Fight with all you've got!!!

E) "Adversity reveals the man to himself." How are you doing?

THE ESSENCE OF SUCCESS

1) Know exactly what you want.
2) Find the right mate.
3) Write down your goals without limit.
4) Make a plan for achieving all your goals and dreams.
5) Work with and associate with successful people.
6) Know the money.
7) Take action, take responsibility and never quit.
8) If your plan is not working, change it immediately.